Sick and Tired of Feeling Sick and Tired

Living with Invisible Chronic Illness

Dedicated
to
our parents

Michael and Mary   *William and Cecelia*

Contents

Preface

The French writer Gustav Flaubert said that we do not choose our subjects for writing, they choose us. This book certainly chose us. Mary had been traveling the arduous path to diagnosis and treatment for her multiple sclerosis. She was hearing from her clients and from others similar stories of the struggle that chronic illness poses; she was beginning to consider the challenge of writing about what she and they were confronting. Paul had been wrestling with the desire to write—a desire prodded by the question asked of him at the end of talks he had delivered or workshops that he had conducted: "Have you written any of this?"

As we talked of our individual plans to write, the idea of collaboration emerged. Together we would try to communicate what we were each wanting to express. We would attempt to apply to the challenge of coping with chronic illness the convictions that we share—that the communication skills which promote real meeting can be learned, that we can become aware of and change the way that we talk to ourselves, that we can form images of hope that will direct our lives creatively, that we can alter the stories that we live by to make them more congruent with reality, and that we can grow to be more authentically and peacefully ourselves.

We decided to direct our book to people plagued with chronic illness and to the people with whom they relate—

spouses, family members, friends, colleagues, and employers. We particularly hope that physicians, psychologists, and
all other health–care providers will read the book, since people with chronic illness are so dependent upon their understanding and support.

We hope that the resulting book will inform, nourish,
and encourage you who are suffering with invisible chronic
illness. We hope that you will be inspired to trust yourself
and your personal experience, that you will treat yourself
with gentleness and grow in appreciation of your unique-
ness. We hope that you will be encouraged to express your
needs with greater freedom. We hope that you will grow in
understanding for those who love you and learn to meet
them more wisely.

Thank you for taking us into your lives.

Acknowledgments

It is a pleasure to have the opportunity to express in writing our thanks to the many generous people who have helped to make this book possible.

First of all, we are especially indebted to Dr. John Balistreri, who read and reread the work as it progressed and offered invaluable advice as to style and content. We thank our typist, Virginia Menz, who met every deadline with skill and warmth. We are grateful to all of the associations of the illnesses discussed in the book for their encouragement and for the information that they provided—we note particularly Mary Lou Ballweg, President of the Endometriosis Association, John Huber, Executive Director of the Lupus Foundation of America, Micelle E. Vilk, Administrator of the Endometriosis/Data Project, and Betty Fairbanks, Executive Director, and staff Marilyn Kirchner and Carol Palumbo of the Western Connecticut Chapter of the National Multiple Sclerosis Society. We owe thanks to all of the doctors who gave of their time and experience in interviews with us. We deeply appreciate Dr. James Crane's competent and caring attention.

So many people assisted us with ideas and buoyed us with their enthusiasm that a full list would be voluminous. We are delighted to mention Susan Earle, Marilyn Gates Hart, and Rosalie Berkowitz. We thank the Ferguson Library in

Stamford, Connecticut, for its excellent facilities and efficient staff. We are grateful to our astute editor, Susan Barrows Munro, for her prompt and insightful assistance. We thank Ruth Wreschner, Joan Bossert and Ross and Eleanor Millhiser for their generous help. We are very, very appreciative to our families and to our colleagues at Touchstone: Communication for Effective Meeting, particularly to Dennis and Rita Shaughnessy for all their support and interest. And we are indebted to Carol Look who proofread the galleys with painstaking care.

It is to our clients and the people we interviewed whose lives are reflected in the book that we are most grateful. Their names and the details about the circumstances of their lives have been changed to protect their anonymity. They are a constant source of inspiration to us. We are profoundly grateful for their trust, their courage, and their goodness. This book is about them and for them and for all others like them who struggle to cope with illness and adversity.

I

The Experience of Invisible Chronic Illness (ICI)

Damage to the body causes diminution of the self, which is further magnified by debasement by others.

Robert F. Murphy

1

Introduction to Invisible Chronic Illness

"I want to be well. I'm willing to fight, but . . ." "But what?" Dr. Diamond asked. "But I must know what I'm fighting. I must have a name for this illness of mine."

Henrietta Aladjem

Recently, returning to Stamford, Connecticut, from a talk in New York, we turned off the highway behind a young man on a motorcycle. As we entered an intersection on a local street, the cyclist suddenly skidded and, in attempting to right his vehicle, spun out of control. We pulled over immediately and rushed to his still form. Within seconds, we were joined by other motorists who had pulled to the side. Some of us held his hands and murmured soothing words, others gathered his wallet, keys, and coins and carefully placed them in a pile next to him. Another person ran to a phone booth at a nearby gas station to call the police. In the space of a few minutes, all our efforts were employed unquestioningly to care for this young man. Later, we reflected on the fact that, faced with such evident disaster, we all responded, as if by instinct, to the needs of the young motorcyclist. Our own needs to get home to rest after a long day or to reach an appointment on time were temporarily suspended in favor of our concern for the cyclist.

The human potential to reach out in care seems to be tapped particularly when the need of the other is indisputably apparent. National disasters, such as the earthquake in Armenia in 1989, inspired an international outpouring of aid in the form of technological and medical assistance, despite the more typically felt restrictions of ideological differences between nations. The deep, instinctual, human capacity to act compassionately when confronted with disaster can overcome the powerful pull of skepticism, anger, or hate.

What happens to this human reaction when the crisis of the person is not as patently clear as we witnessed in the fallen motorcyclist? When, for example, a man stumbles in front of us, we may start to wonder, "Is the person about to fall? Has he drunk too much? Is this just a momentary loss of balance?" Once we start to puzzle over the reason, we hesitate. "Does this person need my help? Did he do something that he shouldn't have that caused his stumble? Is he fine?" Unsure as to the cause of the stumble, we are less likely to move swiftly into action than if the person did, for instance, actually faint. And if we suspect that he has brought his problem on himself by doing something foolhardy or inappropriate, we may become judgmental and refuse to provide help even if requested. In our hesitation, we may begin to feel self-protective, "Will I be rejected if I offer help? Will I risk being hurt physically? What if the person resents my offer of help and regards it as an insult?" Such reflection diminishes the immediate impulse to provide care for the other.

The dilemma described above is at the heart of the distress felt by millions of people who suffer from invisible chronic illnesses (ICI), that is, diseases that are characterized by chronicity and symptoms that are not externally manifested. Symptoms common to invisible illnesses are chronic fatigue, chronic pain, memory loss, transient vision disturbances, muscle weakness, bladder urgency, peculiar physical sensations (numbness, tingling, "pins and needles," hot flashes), skin irritation, intestinal distress, and cognitive difficulty. These symptoms do not show up in a way that makes it obvious to an observer that a person is suffering. Unlike a wound that bleeds or requires stitches, a mending limb that is encased in a cast, or malfunctioning legs that necessitate use of a wheelchair, the symptoms of invisible illnesses have no external evidence of suffering that elicit compassion. Instead, the patient often endures suspicion and withdrawal from others. And so, in addition to disturbing, even agonizing and disabling symptoms, the patient of invisible illness suffers, often deeply, from the negative reactions of others. Such reactions frequently lead the patient to confusion, loneliness, self-pity, and self-doubt.

A patient, Anna, who is suffering from fibromyalgia, a condition that causes chronic pain, related this incident to us:

> I was standing on line at the passport agency. The room was very warm and the wait seemed interminable. I thought at one point that we had been standing for fifteen minutes without any turnover at the counter. The pain traveling across my shoulder and down my right arm was excruciating. Childishly, I wanted to lean my head on the man in front of me. I wanted to cry or throw a tantrum and toss my papers on the floor. I considered approaching the agents to tell them that I needed special assistance. But I felt reluctant, wondering what I would tell them. If I said, "I'm in pain so hurry me through," you can imagine the look I would get. I even fantasized about going up and saying, "I have cancer and I'm dying. Can you speed up the process?"
>
> In the middle of these thoughts, a man in a wheelchair entered the stuffy room looking lost. A passport agent went to his side and bent towards him. They spoke for a few minutes. Then she brought him forms and completed them for him. She gathered their completed work up in her hands and took them with her and disappeared behind the counter. She returned shortly with papers in hand. They exchanged a few words again, he signed the papers, and then turned his wheelchair towards the exit, which the agent opened, and left.
>
> I felt tears of frustration spill down my face. I had been standing in utter pain for thirty minutes and contemplated a possible twenty more. For the millionth time

since I have had to deal with this condition, I "wished" that I bore some sign that revealed the suffering I am enduring and then maybe others would assist me as the passport agent had helped the man in the wheelchair.

Then I felt small and selfish for having those thoughts. God knows, I don't want to be disfigured or incapable of walking. And believe me, I didn't begrudge for a second the help that the man in the wheelchair had received. I was even impressed by and admiring of the agent who had, of her own accord, gone out of her way to make obtaining a passport as easy as possible for him. But, oh, how I resented this disease that makes me suffer so terribly and restricts my life, at the same time that no one can see the suffering and no one offers help.

Anna's experience at the passport agency typifies the stressful consequences of chronic invisible illnesses. Diseases such as chronic fatigue syndrome, irritable bowel syndrome, HIV infection, multiple sclerosis (MS), endometriosis, Crohn's disease, fibromyalgia, and lupus erythematosus, though vastly different illnesses, share characteristics that encompass invisible illness. They are diseases that cause extraordinary pain, fatigue, and a multiplicity of other symptoms that result in great distress and disability. These symptoms may seem to be the kind that most of us feel from time to time. Pain, for example, is part of everyone's life. We feel it with a minor sunburn, a stubbed toe, a bruise, or a hangnail. We feel it more intensely from a broken limb, from a third degree burn, or after surgery. It is part of an inborn warning system that notifies us that something needs to be tended to, whether with rest, medication, or a band-aid. For the most part, when the cause of pain is removed or when a recuperative period is over, the pain lessens and eventually retreats completely.

For chronic pain sufferers, however, there is rarely sufficient relief from pain and always the threat of a lifetime of pain—pain more intense than any caused by the bumps and bruises of a normal life. It may be as intense as that which is experienced after surgery but without any promise of relief. The quality of this pain is so different from transient aches and pains that language is inadequate to the task of describing it.

Similarly, fatigue is a symptom of some of these illnesses. At some point in the day, we all feel tired. We feel tired when we work too hard, don't sleep at night, or exercise too vigorously. There are myriad reasons for feeling tired. Like pain, tiredness is ordinarily the body's means of telling us that it is time to rest. Fatigue for those with chronic illnesses, however, can actually be disabling. This fatigue is relentless. Overexercise or overwork does not cause it and bed rest frequently fails to relieve it. It appears regardless of activity or inactivity, happiness or sadness. It simply exists in and of itself, and no medication, positive thought, or rest can relieve it.

Nonmeasurable Symptoms

Symptoms of invisible chronic illnesses are not only non-observable, but also typically immeasurable. They are subjective experiences. Thus, if a person who is suffering from multiple sclerosis notes that his memory seems to be lacking, there are few measures to determine whether indeed his ability to remember is failing. If someone cannot remember his name, family, or occupation, we acknowledge a serious and evident condition of amnesia. But when the memory loss is subtle and transient, we must rely on the person's self-awareness and description of the impairment. The person's subjective experience, however, is one that the patient, his family, and health-care providers reluctantly trust. The patient may wonder, "Is this really happening or am I just tired?" The patient's wife may reflect, "He always forgets at the most inopportune times, like when he is supposed to pick up a few groceries." The doctor may muse, "This patient is under too much stress." Without proof of a deficiency, such as results of medical tests, everyone seems bent on disproving the possibility that there has indeed been memory loss—the patient because he is self-doubting, the family members because they are suspicious, frustrated, or frightened, and the doctor because he doesn't observe any perceptible problem.

James, who has "mild" multiple sclerosis, describes a typical experience of what it is like to have a problem that is experienced but cannot be proven:

> I have been playing golf for fifteen years, and every Saturday in the past few years I have played with three buddies of mine. We wager on each hole. Lately, when we finish a hole and I try to count my strokes, I can't remember a thing. It's weird. No matter what I do, I just can't remember the strokes. At first, we all laughed— joked about getting older. But after a while my partner was getting pissed off. My forgetting was interfering with our game. Once we gave up a hole because I just couldn't be sure about a stroke. We've figured out a way to keep count, but it's embarrassing and it isn't funny anymore. It is strangely happening at other times too. Like I'll watch a news program and my wife will ask about a news item that I've just seen and I'll be completely blank. I can't remember a sequence of information. I can remember the last part—strange.
>
> I have this sickening sensation in my stomach as I strain to remember. I try to remember rather than just admit to myself that I can't and then relax.
>
> I was so disturbed that I went to the neurologist. He asked me to describe my memory problems and when I was finished he chuckled a bit and said, "You know, Jim, we are all getting older—you probably have to start keeping lists." When I told him that I had done some reading about multiple sclerosis and memory loss as a common symptom, he said, "So they say, so they say. But I don't think so. The researchers keep debating the issue. You just have to make sure that you are getting enough rest. Who knows, it may be that your limp so distracts you when you are playing that you lose some

of your concentration." I felt foolish when I left the office. I felt like I would have to argue with him to get him to understand that I really had a problem. But I figured it wasn't worth the bother since there wasn't anything he could do for me anyway.

But I would have liked to have been able to tell my wife, "The neurologist confirmed that something is wrong with my memory." She wants to understand, but she thinks I've always been absentminded and now I'm even more so. I'm not sure why I need anyone else to acknowledge what is happening to me. I feel furious when it happens. I guess I want to prove that it's really happening.

Diagnostic Dilemma

Jim's frustration with the immeasurability of his memory loss illustrates another integral aspect of the phenomenon of chronic invisible illnesses. Invisible diseases are so difficult to diagnose that they tend to be identified by the process of eliminating other disease possibilities. Patients become aware of vague, sometimes transient symptoms. Multiple sclerosis, for example, may appear initially as numbness in the limbs. The patient may dismiss the symptom as a result of excessive exercise; when he changes his exercise routine and the numbness passes, he is convinced that the new regimen relieved the problem. Then a new symptom occurs, such as intense fatigue, and the patient may feel compelled to see a physician.

Once the patient visits the physician, both he and the physician are confronted with the task of identifying the underlying cause of the symptom. Identifying the source is complicated by the type of symptoms that are described— numbness, fatigue, vision disturbance, pain. These symptoms defy medical measurement. They appear to be vague and unrelated. A persistent patient and a responsible doctor face the challenging prospect of determining the causes of the symptoms through the process of eliminating one possibility after another. The process is anxiety-provoking, uncomfortable, time-consuming, and costly. Doctor and patient struggle with the suspicion that the symptoms are psychosomatic or that the patient suffers from a mental disturbance. With each visit to the doctor and each test, the patient becomes hopeful that, at last, he will have an answer. Fear and dread of having a serious illness are surpassed by the driving need to know "What is making me so miserable?" This need to know is associated with the belief that "Once I know what I have, then I can handle it and receive treatment that will make me feel better, and I'll know that I'm not crazy."

Unfortunately, for patients with ICI, the diagnosis brings short-lived relief. The fear that the disease will attack vital organs, as, for example, in lupus or multiple sclerosis, replaces the relief felt on hearing the diagnosis. The diagnosis of post-polio syndrome triggers terrifying reminders of illness. For patients who are diagnosed with chronic fatigue syndrome, irritable bowel syndrome, or fibromyalgia, there is the disturbing fear that the disease has not been accurately identified. One patient cried, "How can I feel this awful and have something as vague and untreatable as irritable bowel syndrome? I am so afraid that someday they'll find that I have cancer, but then it will be too late."

Ellen's experience is typical of a diagnosis built upon a bewildering process of elimination:

> A year and a half ago, I started feeling this pain in my hand and somewhat in my shoulder and arm. I was pretty sure that the pain was caused by this new weight-lifting program I was doing. So I stopped for a while, but it got worse anyway. They thought at first that I had something called carpal tunnel syndrome. One doctor wanted to operate right away, but another advised me to wait. Now they are sure that it isn't carpal tunnel, but they aren't sure what it is. This last year the pain has gotten worse all the time. It is mostly in my neck, shoulder, and left arm. It has gotten so bad that I had to

quit my job. I can't concentrate or complete anything. Sometimes I wish I could just die, I am so overwhelmed with the pain.

I think I've had every test you can think of: MRI, EKG, EEG, spinal tap, X-rays, blood test, and urine tests. I've tried so many medications that my bathroom shelves look like a pharmacy. I decided to stop taking some narcotic pain relievers because I was afraid of the side effects, but I went through horrible withdrawal that was almost as bad as the pain. I've tried physical therapy, hypnotherapy, homeopathy, and biofeedback. They helped a little. Some of the medications helped somewhat too. But I'm still in pain.

And—this is what is so unbelievable to me—I still don't know what I have. They have kind of reached a consensus that it is fibromyalgia, but one doctor said he doesn't even believe that there is such a condition. He said it is just a "catch-all" term that is used when there is no other explanation.

When Ellen first told us her "story," she felt sure that her experience was unique. She was startled but comforted by the realization that she was not alone in her quest to find a name for her illness and a means of coping with it. For those of you reading this book who recognize the experience of illness that we have described, we hope that the following chapters comfort you and inspire you to live with your illness in a way that gives you dignity, confidence, and hope.

2

The Baffling Forms of ICI

Man's pursuit of happiness is
fraught with tragedy.

Mortimer Adler

The experiences that Jim, Anna, and Ellen describe in Chapter 1 reveal the distressing facets that typify invisible chronic illnesses. ICIs are characterized by a series of symptoms that are disturbing, disabling, and seemingly unrelated. They are particularly difficult to measure and tend to defy identification by medical tests. They are, as a result, difficult to diagnose. The person is sentenced to days, months, even years of distress without clear-cut knowledge of what she suffers. She may look "well," but such appearances hurt not only others' but also her own ability to trust that a problem indeed exists. The chronic nature of these diseases threatens to produce a lifetime of unwellness. There is always the possibility that the disease may worsen to cause grave incapacitation, yet there is the equal possibility that the disease may go into remission. The constants are uncertainty and fear. The torturing hope/fear that "this is all imagined" or "psychological" is ever present.

There may be many illnesses that are difficult to diagnose and that fit the ICI definition (for example, allergies, hypoglycemia, mitral valve prolapse, depression, scleroderma). We have identified fourteen that exemplify the condition. Brief descriptions follow.

Charcot-Marie-Tooth disease (CMT)
Chronic fatigue syndrome (CFS)
Endometriosis
Fibromyalgia
HIV infection
Inflammatory bowel diseases
   Colitis
   Crohn's disease
Irritable bowel syndrome (IBS)
Lupus erythematosus (lupus)
Lyme disease
Migraine headaches
Multiple sclerosis (MS)
Post-polio syndrome
Premenstrual syndrome (PMS)
Thyroid disease

ICIs share these characteristics:

- Nonobservable symptoms, for example:
  Pain
  Fatigue
  Bladder urgency
  Vision disturbance
  Cognitive difficulty
  Memory loss
  Muscle weakness
  Incoordination
  Lack of balance
  Constipation
  Diarrhea
  Intestinal distress
  Unusual physical sensations—numbness, tingling, hot and cold flashes
  Skin irritations—itching, rashes
  Sleep disorders
  Headaches

- Many of the symptoms in milder forms are part of life—e.g., pain—and in more extreme forms are difficult to describe adequately.
- Some symptoms (pain, fatigue, menstrual pain, diarrhea, constipation, incontinence) have a social stigma attached to them, which causes the patient to believe it is "socially unacceptable" to talk about them.
- The symptoms tend to be immeasurable. The degree of subjective pain and fatigue, for example, cannot be measured objectively.
- The patient tends to look well and has even learned, out of necessity, to appear "as if" everything were fine.
- Invisible chronic illnesses are difficult to diagnose. For example, many of the initial symptoms of multiple sclerosis, such as fatigue and vision disturbance, may represent a multitude of illnesses, including mental illness.
- The diseases are chronic, in other words, they do not follow the typical progression of illness: (1) onset, (2) period of illness, (3) recuperation, (4) recovery.
- There are no cures for invisible chronic illnesses.
- The disease is marked by periods of exacerbation and remission. At times, the patient may feel well—free from symptoms—only to relapse.
- Due to complications of diagnosis, the patient frequently endures the suspicion of others, as well as her own suspicions, that the condition is psychological.
- A constant threat exists that the patient will enter a completely debilitating stage. Even if the disease is in remission, the threat of a relapse from which the patient will never recover is always present.
- Treatments vary in effectiveness.

Description of Invisible Chronic Illnesses

CHARCOT-MARIE-TOOTH DISEASE

What Is It?   Charcot-Marie-Tooth disease (also known as hereditary motorsensory neuropathy and peroneal muscular atrophy) is a hereditary disorder of the peripheral nervous system. Slow degeneration of the nerves causes impairment of normal use of legs, arms, and hands. The result of nerve degeneration is muscle wasting. Sensory perception is affected, making it difficult to feel hot and cold in the body's extremities. Fine movement of the hands, such as in writing, becomes increasingly difficult for some people. A high arched foot is one of the first signs of the presence of CMT. Symptoms include the arched foot, diminished sense of touch, pes cavus foot (foot drop and hammer toes), and in some cases chronic pain and fatigue. CMT is classified as Type I or Type II. In general, the two types are similar in presentation; they differ in nerve conduction velocities (speed with which messages are communicated in the peripheral nervous system). The severity of illness varies widely, even within the same family, although men tend to suffer more severe disability than women. People with CMT typically have a normal life span.

Who Gets It?   Men, women, and children are afflicted with CMT. It is inherited in an autosomal dominant pattern. In other words, there is a 50 percent chance that the illness will be passed on if one parent has the disease. Carrying the CMT trait does not predictably lead to the onset of symptoms. Approximately 125,000 people in the United States are diagnosed with CMT.

CHRONIC FATIGUE IMMUNE DYSFUNCTION SYNDROME (CFIDS)

What Is It?   Chronic fatigue immune dysfunction syndrome (CFIDS) is also referred to as chronic fatigue syndrome (CFS), chronic infectious mononucleosis, myalgic encephalomyelitis (ME) in England, Canada, New Zealand, and Australia. It has been derogatorily called "yuppie flu." Research suggests that CFIDS is an immune dysfunction disorder triggered by a viral illness. The outstanding symptom of CFIDS is chronic fatigue. Fatigue, however, is only one of a complex constellation of symptoms, which include swollen and painful lymph glands, sleep disturbance, headaches, cognitive impairment (memory loss, confusion, decrease in ability to concentrate), and low-grade fever. Symptoms wax and wane (exacerbate and remit); typically they eventually plateau. They may clear up in six months or persist for years. CFIDS does not result in death. In some instances people with CFIDS spontaneously recover. The Centers for Disease Control (CDC) have produced a provisional "working case definition" of CFIDS to guide physicians in the diagnosis of this illness. It is noted in "The CFIDS Chronicle,"[1]

> Unfortunately, many physicians are not very familiar with CFIDS and have difficulty diagnosing it. Others still do not even know that the illness exists or have only recently learned of it. As a result, people with CFIDS have often been misdiagnosed in the past and many still are, sometimes as having a psychosomatic or affective disorder because such conditions are also diagnosed by exclusion in many cases.

As yet, there is no conclusive evidence of a specific cause of CFIDS; thus, there is no lab test to identify the marker of CFIDS in the body. Fortunately, research on CFIDS has proliferated since the identification by Dr. Paul Cheney and Dr. Daniel Peterson of an unusual number of cases in a small town in Nevada. Retroviruses, herpes virus, and enteroviruses are being investigated as triggers of the immune dysfunction of CFIDS. Researchers are also examining the sluggish action of cytoxic T-cells (killer cells of the immune system that attack anything foreign that enters the body). Some researchers suspect a fungal trigger of CFIDS.

Who Gets It?   Women are more typically affected by CFIDS than men, though both sexes are susceptible to the illness. People tend to contract the illness between the ages of twenty and forty. Dr. David Bell, a physician in New York, has identified the syndrome in children.

ENDOMETRIOSIS (ENDO)

What Is It?   Endometriosis is a disease that involves endometrium, the tissue that lines the uterus. Normally, this tissue builds up only in the uterus and is shed each month during menstruation. In women who have endometriosis, the endometrium also implants itself outside the uterus. The abnormal (ectopic) growths of endometrium can be found almost anywhere in the body but are typically found in the fallopian tubes, ovaries, bowel, bladder, and outer surface of the uterus. Not as usual are growths outside the abdominal cavity, such as in the rectum, external genitals, lungs, arms, legs, and thighs. During the menstrual cycle, as the endometrium increases in the uterine cavity, the ectopic growths also build up outside the uterus. While the endometrium lining is eliminated from the uterus, these growths have no way of shedding the blood. The result is inflammation of the surrounding tissue and scar formation. If the growths are large, they can rupture or cause blockage in the bladder and bowel.

As with the other ICIs, the symptoms of endometriosis vary in kind and intensity from woman to woman. The symptoms include painful menstruation, painful intercourse, chronic pain (in the back, legs, gastrointestinal tract, and urinary tract), heavy and irregular bleeding, chronic fatigue, and infertility.

The cause of endometriosis is unknown. A number of theories proposed and under investigation include a genetic predisposition for the disease and the possibility that remains from the embryotic stage develop later in adulthood into endometrium. The most widely held theory as to the cause of the illness is retrograde flow, that is, endometrial tissue that is shed through the fallopian tubes and deposited into the pelvis. This theory, however, does not explain the mechanism of endometriosis fully, since some women with retrograde flow do not develop endometriosis. Some researchers suggest that a dysfunction of the immune system may be involved in endometriosis.

Endometriosis is a benign (nonlifethreatening) disease. It cannot be cured but it can be clearly diagnosed with tests, and there are treatments that can relieve the intensity of symptoms. Ignorance in the general and medical population is an additional battle that women who suffer with endometriosis must confront. The suspicion that the disease is psychosomatic is lessening, but slowly. A psychologist, Mary Lou Hollis, reflects this ignorance in the conclusions of her study. "Endometriosis is a nice protection for some women who do not want to have children," and "The endometriotic woman is non-assertive and conforms to social expectation."[2]

Who Gets It?   Endometriosis afflicts about five million American women during their reproductive years—late teens through their forties. It strikes women of all races and socioeconomic levels.

FIBROMYALGIA (FM)

What Is It?   Fibromyalgia is a musculoskeletal condition that is sometimes referred to as fibrositis, myofibrositis, fibromyositis, and myofascial pain syndrome. It is characterized by the presence of diffuse and persistent pain and chronic fatigue. Sleep disturbance is another common symptom. Sleep disorders that affect people with fibromyalgia are myoclonus (spasms in legs and arms at night), alpha-delta sleep disruption (delta sleep disrupted by alpha waves), and nonrestorative sleep (waking after sleep with stiffness and soreness). Less common symptoms are frequent headaches, dry eyes, hair loss, sun sensitivity, and irritable bowel syndrome. Symptoms tend to fluctuate and do not necessarily occur simultaneously. They may appear slowly or attack suddenly.

Although fibromyalgia may have been a condition plaguing mankind forever, it has only recently been given serious attention by the medical and research communities. Research in the 1980s and 1990s proliferated and suggested a basis for diagnosis. Fibromyalgia may be identified when patients report a history of pain over an extended period of time in eleven out of eighteen specific tender points. Tender points are zones of the body that when palpated (pressed) are excruciatingly painful. For many people with fibromyalgia, sleep is not restful. The symptoms of fibromyalgia are so similar to those of chronic fatigue syndrome that some researchers believe that they "are different strains of the same disorder."[3] They do differ, however, in that "CFS patients have greater fatigue while FM patients have greater pain."[4] There are no cures for fibromyalgia, but some symptoms can be treated.

The cause of fibromyalgia, as with all ICIs, is unknown. Some areas of possible cause that are being investigated are central nervous system abnormalities, viral triggers of FM such as human-herpes-6 virus, rubella, human T-cell lymphotropic virus (HTLV), head and neck trauma, bacterial infection, low-level amino acids, and metabolic disturbances.

Who Gets It?   Primarily women suffer with fibromyalgia. It may be that more women than men are diagnosed with fibromyalgia because women, in general, tend to seek medical attention more often than men. There may be, however, a link between fibromyalgia and hormones, since there appears to be an increase in flare-ups of symptoms before menstruation. Evidently, this does not explain the instances of fibromyalgia that have been found in children and men.

HUMAN IMMUNODEFICIENCY VIRUS (HIV)

What Is It?   Human immunodeficiency virus is the most widely accepted cause of acquired immune deficiency syndrome (AIDS). When a person is infected with HIV, the potential for AIDS and AIDS-related complex (ARC) is ever present. We are primarily focusing on the HIV stage of AIDS since that condition is characterized by the invisible chronic illness factors. First of all, it is not possible to detect from casual observation that a person has HIV. Someone with HIV generally appears healthy. People with HIV face the inevitable progression of the illness and development of AIDS, but the illness develops in different patterns and the nature and severity of the symptoms are different for each person.

Symptoms that may occur in the early stages of infection include fever, fatigue, tender and swollen lymph glands, and headaches. Often these symptoms temporarily recede. When the disease becomes more active, new symptoms occur, such as chronic diarrhea, chronic fatigue, weight loss, cognitive changes, skin disease, night sweats, lymphoma, and ear-nose-throat problems. HIV sufferers can experience years of exacerbations and remissions of these symptoms. Early recognition is vital for treatment and relief of the symptoms and to assure longer survival. Opportunistic infections (infections that the healthy immune system routinely wards off) eventually weaken the immune system, allowing the onset of AIDS.

Who Gets It?   The early cases of diagnosed AIDS in the United States were found in 1981 in Los Angeles and New York. During the early and middle 1980s AIDS was particularly found in the homosexual, Haitian, and hemophiliac populations. Since that time, AIDS has been discovered in the heterosexual population, particularly among intravenous drug users and their sex partners. Men, women, and children are vulnerable to HIV infection. No race appears to be exempt.

INFLAMMATORY BOWEL DISEASE (IBD)

What Is It?   Included in the inflammatory bowel disease category are two diseases, Crohn's disease and ulcerative colitis. Crohn's disease, also referred to as ileitis and regional enteritis, is an inflammatory disease that causes thickening of tissue in the small intestine (ilieum) and colon. The thickening can cause obstruction in these organs. Fistulae (inflamed connections) are formed when the inflammation spreads to the bladder and other parts of the bowel. Ulcerative colitis attacks the colon (the last section of the large intestine) and the rectum. Onset of colitis is marked by soft and loose stools (more so than usual) mixed with blood and a pressing sensation that signals an intense need to defecate (tenesmus).

Symptoms common to inflammatory bowel disease are diarrhea, loss of appetite, weight loss, abdominal pain, and rectal bleeding. Severe cases of these two diseases can cause systemic symptoms; in other words, other systems of the body are affected, such as the liver, skin, joints, and eyes.

Inflammatory bowel diseases are characterized by ICI conditions. Authors of *The Crohn's Disease and Ulcerative Colitis Fact Book* note, "The diseases are chronic and as yet their cause—and therefore their cure—are unknown. Some people have mild symptoms while others have severe and disabling ones."[5] In either case, symptoms exacerbate and remit. Treatment and surgery can alleviate the intensity of symptoms. Some causative agents being investigated are intestinal bacteria, virus, and dysfunction of the immune system; yet no single lab test identifies the disease.

Who Gets It?   Approximately 500,000 people in the United States have been diagnosed with inflammatory bowel disease. Estimates that include people who suffer with the illnesses but have not been diagnosed may go as high as two million. Males and females are vulnerable to Crohn's disease and colitis. Onset generally begins between the ages of twelve and the late twenties; a less frequent age onset is after the age of fifty. IBDs appear predominantly in developed countries.

IRRITABLE BOWEL SYNDROME (IBS)

What Is It?   Irritable bowel syndrome (erroneously called spastic colon) is the common cold of the intestinal tract.

Elaine Shimberg, author of *Relief from IBS,*[6] estimates that twenty-two million Americans suffer with IBS. Common as it is, IBS makes people feel miserable. This syndrome is a functional disorder; in other words, tests can detect no evidence of pathology to explain the symptoms. Normally, the contents of the intestines are propelled by muscular contractions. In people who have IBS these contractions are irregular and uncoordinated, causing intestinal distress. Symptoms common to IBS are abdominal pain, constipation, diarrhea, alternating constipation and diarrhea, excessive gas, distension and bloating, appetite loss, headaches, and fatigue. Symptoms are aggravated by certain foods, alcohol, caffeine, and smoking. IBS does not lead to cancer or any other disease. Some symptoms can be relieved by changes in diet, eating habits, and medical treatment.

Who Gets It?   In the United States women are twice as likely as men to suffer with IBS. It occurs in young people, with most people identifying the symptoms of the syndrome before the age of thirty-five.

LUPUS ERYTHEMATOSUS (LUPUS)

What Is It?   Lupus erythematosus is an autoimmune disease that generally affects the skin, kidneys, joints, lungs, and blood. It may affect every system of the body. In lupus the immune system becomes hyperactive and produces excessive amounts of the blood proteins called antibodies. When functioning appropriately, these antibodies attack foreign invaders of the body, such as bacteria; during lupus flare-ups, the antibodies attack healthy tissue and cells. Lupus can strike suddenly or appear gradually. Symptoms exacerbate and remit and in some cases may manifest themselves so slightly that they may not be noticed. Symptoms do not occur in a typical pattern, thus complicating diagnosis. One person with lupus may feel flu-like symptoms, while another may have kidney problems. There is no cure for lupus, though symptoms often respond to treatment.

There are three kinds of lupus—discoid, systemic, and drug-induced. Discoid lupus causes a pronounced rash of the face and scalp and severe hair loss (which tends to grow back after flare-up of symptoms) and may leave scars on face and scalp. Typically, discoid lupus causes little internal disease; however, a small percentage (5 percent) of the people with discoid lupus may experience a systemic attack at some time in their lives. Systemic lupus involves not only the skin but also internal systems such as kidneys, blood, joints, tendons, and lungs. Symptoms such as sun sensitivity, pleurisy (sharp pains in lower parts of the chest), joint pain, fever, kidney inflammation, and anemia are common.

The cause of lupus is presently unknown, but intensive research activity takes place worldwide. Some researchers are looking into the possibility that lupus is a viral disease; other causes being investigated are immune dysfunction, sun exposure, and infection.

Who Gets It? Women develop lupus eight to ten times more often than men. The illness tends to attack women during their childbearing years. In some women the first symptoms and signs develop during pregnancy; in others they appear soon after delivery. While men and young children contract lupus less frequently than women, they suffer similar symptoms. The Lupus Foundation of America estimates that there are approximately 500,000 Americans who suffer with lupus.

LYME DISEASE

What Is It? Lyme disease is an inflammatory disorder that it transmitted by a tick-borne spirochete, *Borrelia Burgdorferi*. The disease gained recognition in the United States in 1975, when an unusual number of cases were identified in Lyme, Connecticut—hence the name. Typically, a small red lesion identifies the presence of a tick bite. The symptoms become evident within three to thirty days after the bite's occurrence. They include fatigue, headache, fever, and stiffness of the neck. Less frequently occurring symptoms are backache, nausea, vomiting, sore throat, and swollen lymph glands. When the illness is not detected and treated early, it may trigger neurological problems, arthritis, and persistent muscle pains. Research indicates that Lyme disease may trigger the onset of fibromyalgia. Symptoms may relapse and remit, and they may linger for extended periods of time. Administration of antibiotics is effective treatment once the disease is identified. Diana Benzaia notes, "One of the biggest problems in diagnosing Lyme disease is thinking of it in the first place."[7]

Who Gets It?   Adults and children are susceptible to Lyme disease. Cases of the disease have been noted in almost every state as well as in Europe.

MIGRAINE

What Is It?   Migraine is not, as several individuals vehemently told us, "just a headache." The pain of migraine, a disorder of the cranial circulation, is caused by dilation of the scalp arteries. What causes the dilation is not known, but research suggests that it may be genetically transmitted. Recurrent attacks of intense pain can occur once a day or once a month. The pain may occur unilaterally (on one side of the head) or generally about the head. It often begins in the eye or in the area surrounding the eye. While intensity, type, and pattern of migraine vary from person to person, the symptoms (in addition to dreadful pain) include nausea, vomiting, photophobia (sensitivity to light), and fatigue. Migraine is typically preceded by prodromal symptoms (precursors), which are sometimes called aura symptoms. These symptoms signal the onset of migraine and may include pins and needles in fingers, hands, and face, loss of appetite, irritability, restlessness, and depression. These symptoms abate after the migraine begins.

Who Gets It? Migraine usually begins between the ages of ten and thirty. In some cases migraines go into remission after the age of fifty. Women are more likely than men to be afflicted with migraines (about twice as often); children are struck with the disorder less often than are adults.

MULTIPLE SCLEROSIS (MS)

What Is It? Multiple sclerosis is a disease of the central nervous system in which the nerve cells lose their covering of myelin, a fatty tissue that insulates the cells and facilitates the transmission of messages within the nervous system. Plaques (scars) form where the myelin has been destroyed. These plaques interfere with communication within the nervous system.

The symptoms of MS are multifocal, transient, and recurrent. They include weakness of limbs, bladder urgency, loss of bowel and bladder control, numbness, tingling in limbs, parathesias (shock-like sensations), difficulty of coordination, speech impairment, and chronic fatigue. When MS is suspected from clinical observation, CT scan and magnetic resonance imaging (MRI) can confirm the diagnosis. There is no cure, but some symptoms can be alleviated with treatment.

The course of the disease is unpredictable and varies greatly with each individual. For approximately 20 percent of the population of people with MS the illness is benign. Benign MS is characterized by one or two exacerbations of symptoms with complete recovery. The exacerbations of symptoms may be so mild as to go unnoticed. The majority of people with MS, 60–70 percent, have exacerbating-remitting multiple sclerosis. When an exacerbation of symptoms occurs, it can last for periods of days, weeks, months, or years; then symptoms may remit unpredictably. Remissions may last for extended periods of time, possibly for years. Progressive MS affects 10–20 percent of the MS population. This form of MS appears gradually but steadily progresses and causes incapacitation.

Who Gets It?   Men and women are affected by multiple sclerosis, though it is more common in women between the ages of twenty and fifty. Children under twelve are not susceptible to multiple sclerosis. Perhaps as diagnostic methods become more sophisticated and accurate, the diagnosis of multiple sclerosis may be determined at earlier ages than previously thought. It is typically found in people living in the northern hemisphere. Approximately 250,000 people have been diagnosed with MS in the United States; the National Multiple Sclerosis Society suspects that there may be many more cases of undiagnosed multiple sclerosis.

POST-POLIO SYNDROME (PPS)

What Is It?   PPS, also called post-polio sequelae and progressive post–polio muscular atrophy (PPMA), is regarded as the late effects of polio. In the 1940s and 1950s epidemics of this crippling viral disease caused widespread fear. Vast amounts of money went to support research in search of a cure. The result was the discovery and development of the Salk and Sabin vaccines, which virtually eliminated the disease. But in the 1980s physicians and physical rehabilitation therapists, as well as past victims of polio, observed a consistent set of physical problems being experienced by past victims of polio. Initially, the medical community failed to pay attention to what the polio patients were beginning to call post-polio syndrome. Not until the survivors of polio organized associations such as the Polio Society and the International Polio Network was the syndrome fully acknowledged.

The difference in attention that has been given to polio as opposed to that given to PPS dramatizes the predicament of ICI sufferers. When polio was an evident and widely recognized disease, research was financed and patients were treated with intense medical attention. As an invisible chronic illness, PPS is only beginning to be accepted as an authentic disorder and the victims given the treatment and medical advice they need to manage their symptoms.

The symptoms include fatigue, new joint and muscle pain, decreased stamina, new difficulties in breathing, new muscle weakness, generalized pain, and sensitivity to cold. Not everyone experiences the same symptoms or the same severity of symptoms. According to the Polio Society, "the most widely accepted explanation [for PPS] is that nerve cells damaged by the polio virus decades earlier, as well as the neighboring nerve cells that took over for those killed by the virus, are now wearing out."[8]

Who Gets It?   Approximately 640,000 people contracted polio, and of these it is estimated that half suffer today with post-polio syndrome.

PREMENSTRUAL SYNDROME (PMS)

What Is It?   Premenstrual syndrome is probably the most maligned and dismissed disorder afflicting women. It is characterized by cyclicity, occurring eight to ten days before menstruation and disappearing immediately after menstrual flow begins. Physician and PMS expert Katharina Dalton indicates a specific set of criteria for diagnosis of PMS:

1. Symptoms must be present every month for at least the previous three months.
2. Symptoms must be present premenstrually and cannot start before ovulation.
3. There must be a complete absence of symptoms after menstruation for a minimum of seven days.[9]

The symptoms of PMS are caused by fluctuations in estrogen and progesterone, which cause retention of fluids. Symptoms vary in intensity and nature, but the list includes fatigue, breast swelling and tenderness, weight gain, bloating, headaches, vertigo, abdominal cramps, acne, muscle aches, depression, and irritability. For most women symptoms do not tend to be disabling, but they are disturbing and persistent. For women who suffer with severe PMS the symptoms interfere with normal function and the disorder is agonizing.

Who Gets It?   Millions of women of every race and socio-economic status suffer with this syndrome.

THYROID ILLNESSES

What is it?   Thyroid illnesses are caused by the overproduction of hormone (hyperthyroidism) or the underproduction of hormone (hypothyroidism). These conditions can affect different parts of the body, including the skin, heart, liver, and kidneys. When the thyroid produces too much hormone, primarily triiodothyronine (T_3) and thyroxine (T_4), symptoms such as dry skin, heart palpitations, weight loss, eye complications, bowel dysfunction, and nervousness are triggered. The symptoms caused by an inadequate production of hormone are weight gain, hair loss, prematurely grey hair, fatigue, and constipation.

Hyperthyroidism and hypothyroidism can be detected through blood tests and family history. Unfortunately, people afflicted with these illnesses are often misdiagnosed because such symptoms as fatigue, nervousness, and weight change are indicative of so many illnesses. These conditions can be treated and cured.

Who gets it?   Thyroid illnesses are inherited conditions that are more likely to strike women than men. Hyperthyroidism typically occurs between the ages of twenty and forty while hypothyroidism is more common after the age of fifty.

3

The Psychological Consequences of ICI

It could be said that my illness, although my enemy, is also my ally, my ally in that it removes me from the hustle and bustle and makes me redefine myself. It makes me introspective.

Dennis Potter

ICI can have a devastating impact on the psychic well-being of the individual. No matter how agonizing the physical distress, the mental anguish can be more difficult to bear. Self-doubt, self-loathing, helplessness, powerlessness, anxiety, and fear are some of the demons that victims of ICI battle daily. Invisible diseases can wipe out one's self-confidence and peace and in their place leave painful doubts about one's own sense of what is real.

Self-Doubt

Am I really sick? Am I imagining this? Am I weak? Did I cause this—if I had eaten better or exercised more would I be well today? Am I losing contact with reality?

Anyone who begins each day awakened by pain is convinced that something is wrong with his body. But when he attempts to describe the pain to his physician or to a family member and is met with bafflement or suspicion, he can easily begin to question, "Is it really that bad? Am I imagining it? If I take my mind off it, will it go away? Am I a negative thinker?"

The self-doubt is temporarily dispelled when a new wave of pain overwhelms him or the effect of a pain reliever wears off. Anger frequently accompanies the recurring pain. Anger at self: "I know I am in pain. Why do I doubt myself? Why did I tell the doctor about the pain in such a tentative manner? Why do I always apologize when pain prevents me from participating in activities?" Anger at others: "Why don't they believe me? I resent the implications that I am a hypochondriac. I wish they could feel the pain for just one day when they suggest that I ought to think positively and the pain would go away."

Maureen, a woman who has suffered from endometriosis since she was fifteen, described the self-doubt and anger she has experienced throughout the course of her illness:

> When I first told my mother that I had really bad cramps, she was kind of indifferently sympathetic. She said all women throughout the ages have had to deal with that pain. She said that it's part of being a woman. Then, when I was sixteen, I remember her and my aunt laughing in the kitchen when I was in bed staying home from school because the cramps before my period were so bad. My aunt was saying, "How will she ever survive childbirth?" I remember being so mad I wanted to slap both of them, but I also felt really disgusted with myself. I really wondered if maybe I was a weakling. All my life, my brothers had called me a crybaby. It wasn't until I was in my early twenties that I finally believed enough in myself to begin trying to find out what was causing me so much pain. And even though a gynecologist told me after several years of investigation that I had endometriosis, I am still plagued with the suspicion that I can't take pain. I can still hear my mother saying, "You have to learn how to handle pain better."

Maureen's mother's advice had value to it. Unfortunately, given the admonishing manner in which it was offered and the skepticism behind it, Maureen heard it as confirmation of her own self-doubts. Thus, she spent years of her life in excruciating pain, alternating between doubts about the real cause of her pain and anger at others who didn't believe her.

Maureen's experience is typical of ICI sufferers, whether their symptoms are pain, fatigue, or muscle weakness. They vacillate between conviction that they are truly suffering and doubt that they may be imagining the symptoms or at least the intensity of the symptoms. Or they wonder whether their condition is worthy of real concern. "After all," one woman sadly reflected, "there are a lot of people who have it worse than I do. I mean, people are dying. What right do I have to complain?" Once self-doubts are quelled, victims of ICI can believe for a time in the normalcy of their need for compassion and empathy. They also will feel angry and resentful when they do not receive such responses. On the other hand, when they begin again to doubt that they do indeed have a serious physical problem, they strive to deny the symptoms, "If I put them out of my mind, then they will go away." The doubting individual then sends signals to others—family, friends, physicians—that he does not need attention and care. Such vacillation produces conflict within the person and tension within relationships. Maureen and others like her are at constant war with themselves and their loved ones.

Self-Dislike

How can I look attractive when I am so dependent? Who wants to employ someone who might be ill all the time? Why can't I overcome this illness? If I had greater integrity (more character), I wouldn't be so incapacitated.

Persistent self-doubt results in self-dislike. It is very difficult to feel self-respect and self-affirmation when, in addition to feeling ill, you are overwhelmed with constant misgivings about your condition, especially when these inner doubts are further fueled by the blatant or subtle skepticism of others.

Maureen finds herself struggling between believing in herself and condemning herself for being weak. As we noted in Chapter 1, Jim's self-doubt deprives him of vital energy needed to achieve peaceful acceptance of his condition. Both are left in unpleasant states, angry at themselves and at those around them. They are resentful of the shallow bits of advice they receive from family and physicians, yet they are susceptible to the implied messages that they are weak or aging. They, and thousands like them, live in a lonely, self-doubting, and self-disliking condition.

Uncertainty

Should I have children? Should I get married? Can I go on a trip? Should I register for a course? Should I buy a house with stairs? Is this sensation a new symptom?

"I'm not sure about anything anymore," a client who tested positive to HIV told us. "I'm not even sure of God or why he'd allow me to have this or allow gays to be singled out. I don't know whether to stay in school or whether it makes sense to prepare for the future." The disillusionment and disorientation expressed by this young man are common to many who struggle with ICI. Theologies and life views, self-images and plans for the future are blasted by illness whose effects are very difficult to predict accurately.

Our future, confidently planned for and confidently expected, secures our present. The medical school student, no matter how deeply in debt, is secure in his expectations of a valued and prosperous career. The apprentice pays his dues with the satisfaction of a stable employment for his future. Boot camp is made tolerable by the promise of being a marine. There is no such security-giving anticipation connected to ICI. The sufferers of chronic illness must face an unpredictable course of illness that may allow them to pursue original plans or cause them to be abandoned.

Fear of Mental Illness

Is this all in my head? If I were a more optimistic person, would I feel better? Maybe I just need to lighten up. Am I neurotic or depressed? If I'm not sick, I'm crazy.

Possibly no fear is as harrowing as the fear of insanity. Loss of control is frightening; loss of mental control is terrifying. Our mind is our sense of ourselves and gives us our sense of the world around us. To lose our minds is to lose connection with ourselves and connection with our world. It is to lose the sense that we are in control of what we think, what we feel and how we act. Images of what we would be like without our reason, without our mental faculties, are chilling images of blubbering, incoherent, incontinent unfortunates. Any threat, then, to our rationality is a dire threat to our well-being.

With its baffling symptoms, invisible chronic illness provides precisely such a threat. Symptoms are not only unpredictable but even denied or viewed with suspicion by those we turn to for comfort and support. Henrietta Aladjem, the author of numerous books on lupus and the founder of the Lupus Foundation of America, blames doctors for contributing to this fear of being crazy.

In a conversation with us, this wise woman described the thoughtless manner in which the diagnosis is sometimes given. In her eyes, the doctor rarely communicates awareness of how the diagnosis can affect the patient or the emotional turmoil it will create. He may not take the time to explain the disease, to outline ways of coping, to provide information and options for treatment. In this way he can instill fear; then, unable himself to cope with the patient's emotions, he may refer her to a psychiatrist, confirming her fears of being mentally and emotionally unbalanced.

Irene, a well-informed woman who suffers with CFIDS and endometriosis, spoke about the predicament of people whose symptoms are regarded as psychological problems:

Damaging things get written in our records and we have
no recourse. The Centers for Disease Control specify
that a diagnosis of CFIDS cannot be made if there is a
preexisting psychiatric diagnosis. It seems common sense
to me that if you've been suffering with symptoms for
years, somewhere along the way a psychiatrist or psychologist will have suspected depression or a somato-
form disorder and will have written that diagnosis in
your records.

Fear of the Course of Illness

*Will I always be sick? Will I someday be unable to walk?
Will I need surgery? Will I always be on medication?
Will my family eventually put me in a nursing home?*

Sickness affects not only the body but also the psyche. It
is difficult to feel confident, positive, and cheerful even when
we have just a cold. But we know the cold will pass and so
will our vulnerable sense of self and our dampened spirits.
When we are afflicted with ICI, our body, our psyche, our
whole being is struck down and there is no relief in looking
ahead. In fact, fear of what lies ahead can depress and even
defeat us. On the awful blank slate marked Unknown, we
can inscribe our worst fears: unmitigated pain, total disability, death. With these fears comes mounting anxiety and
even despair.

Giving in to Illness

*How do I combat a disease that is so intangible? What's the
use? Maybe if I get even sicker, then people will see that I am
suffering. Maybe I should let myself go and really look sick. I
would rather die than face this for the rest of my life.*

We all occasionally feel sorry for ourselves. But self-pity
is not attractive; nor is it conducive to a healthy mind-set.

An illogical but frequent effect of being ill is to feel guilt, a sense of being bad. We have heard so many people describe this unpleasant and unfair phenomenon. On some level they feel responsible for their illness. In some way they think that they have not done what they should have done to stay healthy. Maybe it relates to something in childhood that connected having a cold with failing to wear hat and gloves or being nauseated with overeating. Maybe it relates to superstitious beliefs that being handicapped is a curse for sins committed personally or by one's parents. Whatever the cause, for some persons being ill means being guilty or bad.

Meara, a mother of three, has suffered with undiagnosed intestinal problems since she was a young girl and with PMS since the onset of menstruation. She describes the effect of having an undiagnosed condition and PMS.

I've grown up my entire life like I was cursed—not normal—never able to enjoy anything without worrying that I would be sick. Once when I was in camp, when I was a little girl, my intestines flared up every couple of days. Everyone thought I was getting sick to get attention from my counselors. My mother did take me to doctors, but they never found anything wrong. It was never resolved. Do you know, I still struggle trying to believe that it's real even when a doctor tells me it's not in my head.

It is difficult enough to suffer pain and fatigue and their limitations. It is not easy with ICI to feel attractive, upbeat, and included in the active set. But to feel in addition somewhat evil or irresponsible seems like the unkindest cut of all. How can you feel good about yourself if that self is bad?

Roller Coaster Feelings

One minute I'm up, the next I'm down. I feel up when others think I should be down and down when I should be up. What is wrong with me? Why can't I be peaceful or at least settled down?

When a person suffering from ICI is finally diagnosed, the experience is often profoundly relieving. The relief can appear to others as inappropriate. After all, having a major disease is no cause for celebration. But a specific diagnosis is welcome to someone who has struggled with myriad, unobservable, subjective symptoms. Suddenly, with the name of a disease in hand, suspicion from others can be countered. The patient is convinced then that he can confront any accusations of mental instability from others or from within himself with the irrefutable evidence of an identified disease. One patient brought her MRI (magnetic resonance imaging) results to us as if they were a trophy. "Look," she said, "You can see the scars throughout the brain that indicate that I have multiple sclerosis."

The relief is short-lived. Soon the individual is plunged into the fears, frustrations, and discouragements of coping with her illness. One day she suffers excruciating pain and feels despair; the next she has no pain and is euphoric. One morning she feels overwhelming sadness and loneliness; that evening she might feel satisfaction that she has accomplished a great deal. Sometimes guilt overwhelms her at the thought of burdening her family; at other times she enjoys the support of loving relatives. Often she feels hyper; yet again she feels lethargic. Much of the time she feels as helpless in controlling her feelings as she does in controlling her pain.

The physical toll taken by ICI is formidable: relentless fatigue, terrible pain, wearying discomfort. The psychological toll can be exacting. A woman from one of the associations movingly wrote, "For most of us the disease hurts more on the inside (what it does to our hearts, souls, and emotions) than on the outside."[1] Doubts about one's sanity and worth, as well as one's future, can make life a nightmare. Learning to cope with ICI means learning to know oneself. And that learning does not come easily.

4

Three Dimensions of ICI and Their Psychological Impact

'Tis not so deep as a well, nor so wide as a
church door, but 'tis enough, 'twill serve.

Shakespeare

As we were writing the proposal for this book, we talked to each other about our own illnesses. Mary has multiple sclerosis and Paul has suffered from sleep disruption and intestinal problems since he was a child. We were struck by the similarities of our complaints despite the vastly different natures of our illnesses. We both had grappled with symptoms for years, seeking diagnosis and treatment for individual ones. We laughed, somewhat bitterly, as we compiled a list of the diagnoses and treatments that had been suggested to us, the tests we had endured, the physicians we had seen, and the medications we had taken. Our symptoms are different, but both of us experience exacerbation and remission of those symptoms, allowing relief at some times and causing terrible discouragement at others. We both complain of a constant background of unwellness; however, like many people who have invisible chronic illness, we look well.

Despite our common issues around chronic illnesses, we are not affected in the same way and people respond to us differently. Because of multiple sclerosis's potential to cause grave disability, signs of a new exacerbation tend to arouse fear in Mary and protectiveness in those who love her. Paul has struggled with sleeplessness and miserable intestinal distress since his teen-age years. Exacerbations are frequent, and it is rare that a meal is not followed by discomfort. Yet he has never been given a conclusive diagnosis, and although he may suffer physical distress of great intensity, he does not regard his condition as illness. His closest friends express care for him, but not grave concern about his health.

How a person feels about his chronic illness and how people respond to him are influenced by a number of factors that have little to do with the actual effect of the illness on the body. Invisible chronic illnesses share in common the realities that they are chronic and incurable, that they exacerbate and remit, that they resist diagnosis, that they pose a constant threat to physical well-being, and that, while they often leave the sufferer looking well, they exact a physical and psychological toll. But the degree of mental anguish that an individual will suffer from his illness, as well as the amount of care, trust, respect, and compassion he will receive, is dependent upon three factors outside himself:

the social acceptability of the illness;
the clarity of diagnosis;
the potential severity of the illness.

Each of these dimensions can be looked upon as a continuum that runs from negative to positive regarding one ICI relative to other ICIs. Thus, some ICIs are more socially acceptable than others, some yield a clearer or more certain diagnosis, and some are potentially more severe or life-threatening. By isolating and understanding each of these dimensions, sufferers of ICI, as well as those who care for them, can develop a clearer picture of the stresses involved for a particular individual.

The Social Acceptability Factor

Two women are found to have an illness; one has endometriosis and the other has multiple sclerosis. Though each must rise to the challenge of coping with illness, the woman with endometriosis will probably receive less support, since she may feel less freedom to talk about her symptoms of extreme menstrual cramps and painful sex than the woman with multiple sclerosis who is having problems with her vision.

Societal acceptability of an illness and its symptoms ranges widely. At one end of the continuum is HIV infection. The person who finds he has tested HIV-positive probably will not share this knowledge out of fear of utter rejection. Further along the continuum are illnesses such as Crohn's disease, colitis, endometriosis, premenstrual syndrome, and irritable bowel syndrome. Those affected with these illnesses may not fear rejection but their symptoms of nausea, diarrhea, flatulence, or menstrual pain have a stigma attached to them. It is embarrassing to talk about these symptoms, and most people would rather not hear about them.

At the other end of this continuum are illnesses such as post-polio syndrome or Charcot-Marie-Tooth disease. Individuals with these ailments suffer the conditions of ICI but experience little suggestion from society that their illness is repugnant, embarrassing, disgusting, questionable, or sinful. Interestingly, when we did the research and interviews for this book we quickly learned of public figures who have multiple sclerosis (Jimmy Huega) and lupus (Jeremy Dreyfus). Few public figures have openly acknowledged that they have tested positive for HIV, have irritable bowel syndrome, or suffer with endometriosis.

In some ways, no illness is acceptable to society. One person commented to us, "I'd rather be the healthy person in a group than the sick one. I don't mean just because I don't want to feel sick, but also because when you're sick people don't want to be around you." Perhaps he is right. In general, people who are ill cannot contribute much energy to a group, require special attention, have special needs, and draw attention to our human weaknesses. Like the homeless and the newly widowed, the sick present a demand that many feel too inadequate or too embarrassed to meet. Stephanie, a twenty-two-year-old with endometriosis, described an interaction with her brother.

> I knew my brother had been told by our mother that I have endo. She's our conduit of information. One evening my sister-in-law invited me over for dinner. While she was finishing preparing the dinner, my brother and I were in the living room. First we just sat there. The TV was on and he was kind of watching it. Then he said, "So how're you doing?" I was startled but I was pretty sure he meant more than just asking me casually about how the day was. So I said, "I'm doing all right. The pain has been pretty bad but the doctor has given me something to help it." He just looked at me and said, "I'm sorry." He looked so awkward that I kind of mumbled, "It's not too bad." He got up and went to the TV. Turning the volume up he said, "That's good, that's good. I guess things could be worse." I know my brother is uncomfortable talking about practically anything, but I feel sad that he couldn't talk to me at all about something that has so radically affected my life.

Now add to an illness the fact that it cannot be observed. Suppose someone who works with you says he is tired and is absent from work with some frequency. You might easily wonder, "Is he really too tired to work? Is he lazy? Is he a hypochondriac?" If you contemplate such judgments of the person, you are more likely to treat him with criticism and skepticism than with care and compassion. If a person is tired because he has run a marathon, we say, "But of course he is tired." If someone is tired because he is recovering from a bout of pneumonia, we understand the fatigue and act compassionately. Fatigue without an evident cause makes us suspicious; we treat the person with "unsubstantiated" fatigue with distrust.

The person who has chronic pain is frequently treated in a similarly skeptical fashion. American heroes are the strong, silent types who hit home runs, score touchdowns, and rout the enemy, all the time enduring indescribable and unuttered pain. We are supposed to bear with pain and to triumph over it. Pressured by mind–over–body therapies, we are told that we can drive the pain out with positive thoughts. Someone who has chronic pain from migraine, fibromyalgia, back injury, or an unknown source is not only burdened with these messages of stoicism and mind control but must endure distrusting messages from others: "You're inadequate." "You can't take pain." "You're a malingerer." "You ought to feel *this* way."

Women afflicted with endometriosis and premenstrual syndrome have the added burden of symptoms that are taboo subjects. We can just hear Archie Bunker saying, "Aw geez, don't talk about them private female things." No matter how much our society has progressed in regard to sexual issues, we tend to react squeamishly to and disparagingly of "female reproductive" problems. Images of menstruation are not acceptable, and a woman who complains that sex is painful is often regarded as sexually "frigid." The woman with endometriosis endures pain and fatigue. She wrestles with fears regarding treatment options and doubts about being able to bear children. She suffers adverse reactions to medication. Social squeamishness and skepticism add painfully to her list of trials.

A high degree of social unacceptability of an illness can produce an extraordinary impact on the psychological well-being of a person. When we are ill we need the comfort of human sympathy and understanding. If a disease is deemed unacceptable, overtly or covertly, by society, its victims suffer the added burden of isolation and shame. They might even be dissuaded from seeking diagnosis and treatment. Physician Douglas A. Grossman suggests, "Although IBS is the most common chronic gastrointestinal disorder in the Western world, IBS sufferers may be reluctant to acknowledge or seek help for their symptoms and, therefore, may lose the prospect of treatment."[1]

People with irritable bowel syndrome or inflammatory bowel diseases often experience this isolation. Social appropriateness dictates that there are few settings where a person can speak freely about feeling bloated, having excessive gas, feeling constipated, or having a colostomy. One woman who suffered from irritable bowel syndrome said, "I have battled these symptoms for most of my life. They affect my choice of foods, the activities I participate in, my perception of my body, and the kind of work I do. You can see that IBS has affected every part of my life, but I can't talk to anyone about it. No one wants to listen." The avoidance and squirming that greet disclosures about colostomy, for example, are enough to discourage anyone from talking about his fears of ileitis.

People are suspicious and critical of chronic fatigue and chronic pain sufferers, and society frequently imposes a "let's not talk about it" rule on people who have illnesses such as premenstrual syndrome, endometriosis, inflammatory bowel diseases, or irritable bowel syndrome. But an even greater social restriction is levied on people with the HIV virus. We tend to be suspicious of these individuals. "How did you get it?" "What have you been up to?" In addition, we blame and condemn them for their illness. "It's your fault." "It's your punishment for being homosexual or promiscuous or using drugs." Victims of HIV suffer the terror of an illness that may be terminal as well as the ignominy of social scorn and rejection.

Coping with chronic illness is challenging, but it is more tolerable when we can share our fear, self-doubt, anger, or shame with someone else. The more socially unacceptable an illness, the less it is shared. Ironically, when we are scorned, distrusted, and rejected by others, we are prone to attack ourselves with the same attitudes. In our interviews, we found that those patients whose families consistently communi-cated disbelief or disgust about the illness were more apt to feel self-dislike and self-doubt than those patients who were supported by trusting physicians and families.

Clarity of Diagnosis

Every person who has an invisible chronic illness endures a diagnostic process that is exasperating, terribly expensive, and emotionally and physically painful. The ones who receive a clear diagnosis (the sooner the better) have the relative "comfort" of knowing what is causing their symptoms and what they must prepare to face. Others are left to confront the agonizing quandary of a vague diagnosis—or worse, no diagnosis at all. A clear and definite diagnosis of lupus, multiple sclerosis, or Crohn's disease is frightening, but at least awful doubts about being crazy have been dispelled and what seemed like an endless quest for an answer has ceased. Author and president of the Endometriosis Association, Mary Lou Ballweg writes, "Finally, months into this puzzling illness, the laparoscopy was done. Yes, I had endometriosis. Finally, I had a name for my problem."[2]

For someone who has chronic fatigue syndrome, the "comfort" of a diagnosis is often not complete. A person diagnosed with CFIDS, particularly if the fatigue is not accompanied by other outstanding symptoms, may be plagued with an unrelenting concern that the diagnosis is inaccurate. Immobilizing chronic fatigue is difficult enough to bear without the constant worry, "Is this what I really have?" Similarly, migraine sufferers live with the fear that the diagnosis may not be accurate. "Can pain this terrible be 'just' a headache?" "Maybe the pain is a sign of something else, maybe I have a tumor, maybe I am dying."

Almost without exception the people we spoke to wanted a label for their physical complaints. They knew something was wrong with their bodies and they wanted an explanation. Their stories, much like our own, always contained an odyssey in pursuit of diagnosis and treatment. Everyone we spoke to who had been given a diagnosis expressed relief in knowing the illness despite the threat of chronic suffering and little or no treatment. A young woman who has lupus explained to us, "When I would have a very bad attack before I was diagnosed, I would be sure that I was dying. I didn't see how I could feel so sick and not be in mortal danger. Now when I feel sick again, I remind myself that it's lupus. I'm still scared about what may happen to me, but it's not a mystery anymore and I'm not dying." A definite diagnosis not only settles doubt within the person who has the illness and puts an end to much of the doctor and treatment shopping but also puts to rest the doubts of family and friends.

For many of the people who have the illnesses that we have identified as ICI, there is a long period of time—sometimes months or years—before the illness is diagnosed. Imagine the predicament of the person whose initial symptoms are dizziness, headaches, irritability, and lethargy. Not only are these symptoms not measurable, but they are symptomatic of nearly all of the illnesses that we are discussing. Small wonder that physicians find it difficult to arrive at a diagnosis. If this difficulty is a dilemma for the doctor, it is certain agony for the patient. Endless theories are proffered, endless tests administered. Consider some of the conditions that must be ruled out before a diagnosis of multiple sclerosis can be made: "cerebral infarctions, syringomyelia, amyotrophic lateral sclerosis (ALS), syphilis, intervertebral disk, basilar impression, hereditary ataxias, central nervous system tumors, abscesses or other mass legions, vascular malformations of the brain and spinal cord."[3]

We know many people who have endured the diagnostic process, spent a lot of time in hospitals and physicians' offices, emptied their savings accounts, and still not found the explanation for their complaints. Ultimately some of the invisible chronic illnesses can be clearly diagnosed. Blood tests reveal lupus. Laparoscopy can identify endometriosis. Scanning the brain for lesions by magnetic resonance imaging or CT scan and examining cerebral spinal fluid can reveal multiple sclerosis. The trick, sadly, is for the individual to have symptoms severe enough or constant enough to impel the physician to continue the search, prescribe the tests, and examine all of the results. Or the patient must be determined enough and confident enough to keep searching for the doctor who will be thorough. Illnesses such as Charcot-

Marie-Tooth, a rare disease, and post-polio syndrome may not even be considered unless the patient suspects that he has such an illness or an alert physician takes an extensive history of the patient.

People who obtain a diagnosis for their illness can then use the energy that they have put into seeking a diagnosis into learning how to cope with their illness. They can become educated about their illness and understand its typical course, symptoms, and treatments. They can be more informed about the kinds and amounts of foods, activity, and stress that worsen or ameliorate their condition. They can become involved in the associations that disseminate information about their illness and raise funds for research. They can join self-help groups and support groups to feel less alone. They can learn how to talk about their illness and to help others to talk about it. The diagnosis helps to quell self-doubt and suspicion from others while providing the diagnosed with a known adversary.

Is it any wonder that the life of the undiagnosed is filled with anguish? Without an objective explanation of her ailments, the suffering person is terribly vulnerable to the notion that she is suffering from psychosomatic illness or that she is depressed, neurotic, or hysterical. Physician C. Orian Truss argues in his book, *The Missing Diagnosis,* that the labeling of the undiagnosed as hypochondriacs has

> resulted in the heavily disproportionate application of psychiatric methods of treatment in patients whose only psychological problems are those that have been brought on by the failure of the medical profession to correct their long-standing frustrating illness, and by the endless repetition of the medical concept that theirs is an illness related to their own inadequacies.[4]

The person who is not diagnosed and is feeling symptoms such as aches and pains, unusual lethargy, loss of balance, vision disturbance, or skin irritations may toy with the idea that she is crazy but will probably remain convinced that something is wrong with her body. It is important that she voice this conviction, and it is imperative that the doctor take her seriously. Dr. Ellen Idler warns, "Patients who complain of symptoms that medical tests cannot verify should not be dismissed as hypochondriacs. They may be picking up something very meaningful, even if they get a clean bill of health in a physical."[5]

Maybe the physician does trust the patient's experience of her body and the symptoms that she complains of, but he may be as perplexed as the patient as to the cause of the symptoms. A physician's commitment to follow the patient's case is a comfort to the patient, but the patient is still left to cope with the unknown. She usually resorts to self-explanation and experiments with self-treatment. Sometimes her regimen of treatment seems to work so she sticks with it, believing that she has discovered, if not the cause, then surely the cure.

This behavior pattern is reminiscent of B. F. Skinner's learning experiments with pigeons. Some of the birds were given food each time they pecked at a certain lever. They learned that the specific behavior of pecking at the lever would immediately and predictably produce results. Other pigeons were given a pellet of food on an unpredictable schedule that was unrelated to the bird's behavior. These birds developed superstitious-like behavior. They would repeat the sequence of movements (pecking, strutting, turning, head-bobbing) that preceded the arrival of the food, unaware of the irrelevance and impotence of their behavior. People who are trying to cope with an undiagnosed illness speculate constantly and often make connections between their behavior and the waxing and waning of their symptoms that are as inaccurate as the connections made by Skinner's pigeons.

One woman who later learned that she has lupus described her efforts to resolve her first symptoms.

> We were on vacation in Phoenix when I had incredible pain in my joints. It was agony. We were at a resort that had a health center and I went to see the doctor there.

He examined me and said that he thought maybe I had arthritis, but he wasn't sure and he encouraged me to see my doctor when I went home. We were staying at the resort for another week so I tried to figure out what was causing my pain, hoping that I could prevent it. I had been bicycling every afternoon for a couple of hours after lunch. I thought maybe the exercise was hurting me so I stopped the bicycling and read in my room in the afternoon. I started to feel better and by the time I was home in Vermont for several weeks I felt considerably better. I was convinced that the pumping action of riding a bike caused the pain in my joints. So it's funny, so to speak, that I have learned a year later that I have lupus. Probably the hours of incredibly direct and hot Arizona sun caused an exacerbation. The exercise was only a secondary cause of the pain.

Anyone who suffers with illness must listen carefully to physical clues that indicate that something is wrong. She needs to learn what makes her feel better or worse. Essentially, she must learn to trust her own experience. How very hard this is to do, though, when she does not know exactly what illness she is dealing with, when she is plagued with self-doubt, and when some of the people she values most do not trust her.

Having an illness that is inconclusively diagnosed or receiving a diagnosis that many medical professionals dismiss is almost as frustrating as having no diagnosis at all. In a November 1990 *Newsweek* article on CFIDS, the reporter notes that people who suffer from chronic fatigue syndrome in the United States may number in the millions, but you "wouldn't know it to read the mainstream medical journals."[6] CFIDS is particularly representative of all of the baffling ICI conditions. It is truly a puzzling illness for physicians and patients alike. Symptoms of CFIDS vary in intensity and may include "profound or prolonged fatigue, muscle discomfort or myalgia (pain or aching), visual disturbance, psychological problems (anxiety, panic attacks, personality

changes, emotional lability), irritable bowel, and headaches)."[7] Who wouldn't be confused by this baffling array
of vague or unmeasurable symptoms? Who wouldn't confuse this illness with more than one of those we refer to as
ICI? In fact, *The CFIDS Chronicle* notes that the symptoms
of chronic fatigue syndrome "can resemble many disorders,
including mononucleosis, multiple sclerosis, fibromyalgia,
AIDS-related complex (ARC), and autoimmune diseases such
as lupus."[8] Fibromyalgia is often confused with CFIDS. Some
researchers believe that they are the same condition and some
scientists wonder whether fibromyalgia is a condition at all,
as indicated by the title of one article, "Fibrositis, Does It
Exist and Can It Be Treated?"[9]

While debate and research continue, persons who suffer
from these illnesses are burdened with physical symptoms
that are emotionally frightening and discouraging, utterly
confusing, and sometimes completely incapacitating. A discouraged woman said to us after her latest visit to the doctor, "Now they think I have multiple sclerosis. This may
sound sick, but I would rather have MS than CFIDS. It
seems definable." She could have added, "And people will
believe that I am really sick if I can say it's a known disease
that isn't surrounded by debate."

ICI's Potential for Severity

Anyone with ICI lives from day to day with a varying degree
of unwellness. She bears with the exacerbation-remission
cycle, doubts that she can really be helped by physicians,
and wonders what it would be like to feel completely healthy.
But some people with ICI live with the specter of disability
and death. People with HIV infection live daily with the
realization that a symptom—a cold that won't go away or
sudden weight loss—can be a signal of the onset of AIDS,
which at present will in all probability lead to early death.
Many ICIs are not inevitably life-threatening. Colitis, for
example, is not life-threatening, but it does make the person
who suffers from it more vulnerable to cancer than the aver-

age person. On the other end of the severity potential continuum are people with illnesses such as fibromyalgia, migraine, premenstrual syndrome, and irritable bowel syndrome. These people live with discomfort and excruciating pain. They will not, however, have the additional burden of fearing that their life is in danger. People with multiple sclerosis, CMT, and post-polio syndrome may fear the potential of total disability but their illnesses do not pose a threat to life.

People who endure the agonizing symptoms of premenstrual syndrome, endometriosis, chronic fatigue syndrome, irritable bowel syndrome, and migraines might at many times wish to die to escape the pain and discomfort, but they will not die from their illness. Elaine F. Shimberg, author of *Relief from Irritable Bowel Syndrome,* writes,

> IBS does not predispose you to other chronic or life-threatening diseases such as cancer or ulcerative colitis. It will not get worse. You do not require surgery. It is not life-threatening. People don't die from IBS. Unfortunately, you often may feel as though you could die.[10]

Perhaps one of the most wrenching dimensions of these kinds of ICI is the prospect of excruciating, unremitting pain without the relief of cure or death. Physician Katharina Dalton notes, "While accepting that fatalities from the premenstrual syndrome or period pains are rare and the suffering is short-lived, ending with menstruation, nonetheless the suffering, unhappiness and social consequences of it are without limitations."[11]

These illnesses are debilitating and impair normal functioning. Former Detroit Lion Gino Oliveri, for example, has not worked for three years since he contracted chronic fatigue syndrome. He describes the impact of the illness:

> The fatigue, it's deep in my bones. I have five or six eye problems. I get nausea and lymph node swelling throughout my body. I'm confused a lot of the time and

> I have tremendous insomnia. When you've got the flu,
> the first day is bad, but by the fourth day you're back at
> work. I don't see any change at all.[12]

At the critical extreme of the ICI spectrum are those with
HIV infection. The former football player's lament of not
seeing any change at all would be an answer to their pray-
ers. They live day to day, fearing any change that would
signal the beginning of a sickness that might result in death.
At the present time there is no cure for AIDS. Drugs such
as AZT only forestall the onset of illness. Death awaits all
of us; but for those infected with the HIV virus the wait is
predictably short.

Some of the most courageous people we have met are the
young men and women who know that they are HIV positive. Dennis is a twenty-eight-year-old carpenter. For three
years, he and three other carpenters have had their own small
business doing home alterations. Six months ago, Dennis
tested HIV positive. He described to us what the news has
meant to him.

> I dreaded taking the test. I've watched two very good
> friends die of AIDS. I used to think, if I'm HIV positive,
> I don't want to know it. But then I thought, if I am, I
> should know. At first, I wanted to die. I drove to the
> beach and sat by myself most of the day, crying, think-
> ing of what I had wanted in my future, seeing every-
> thing go black. I didn't know if I would tell anyone. It
> started to get dark. I didn't know if I should go home,
> if I should call anyone. I even toyed around with diving
> off the pier. But I finally drove to a good friend's apart-
> ment and we talked all night. Anyway, I joined a sup-
> port group in the city. I've told the guys at work. They've
> been terrific, thank God. I've had to change. I go out
> less. I keep better hours. I eat better. I sure pray more. I
> just have to live as well as I can every day. Maybe there'll
> be a cure; maybe not. I value everything way more than
> I ever did. Most days I'm pretty good.

It has been eye-opening and inspiring to us to counsel those who are HIV positive. Instead of hearing despair, we far more frequently encounter hope, faith, and wisdom. In the face of death, the beauty and value of life seem to be more clearly perceived.

However, the vast majority of those dealing daily with the exigencies of ICI lack the drama of impending death to spark great courage. There is the unremitting, soul-wrenching drudgery of managing pain. The banker with migraines hopes that the blinding pain of his headaches will not prevent him from doing his job. The mother with chronic fatigue prays that her baby sleeps through the night and that a snowfall will not keep the children at home on a school day. The student with irritable bowel syndrome hopes that her bloating and diarrhea do not prevent her from completing a term paper.

There are no societal rituals surrounding ICI: no hospital visits with flowers and sympathy to bestow some degree of validity and importance on the illness and its victim. The individual is on her own to cope with an unending set of painful, bewildering symptoms and the often hurtful reactions of others. The combination of pain and lack of adequate comfort frequently results in depression. Then the depression is blamed for the illness.

Some of the illnesses work directly on the emotions. Premenstrual syndrome is the most evident example of this phenomenon. The syndrome has its own physical dimension of pain and discomfort, but its impact on the emotions can be devastating. Mary Sue is a legal secretary. She came to us after totaling her car in a DWI accident. Only after a number of sessions did Mary Sue begin to talk about her PMS.

> For a week before my period, I'm like somebody else. I don't care about anyone, least of all myself. I fly off the handle. I feel disgusted with myself, with my life. Sometimes I think of killing myself. And, Jesus, if I drink, I go nuts. And during that week it's hard to give a damn

about how much I drink. This week I tore my boss's head off. It's amazing he didn't fire me.

On a severity of illness scale, PMS would seem mild compared to lupus, MS, and chronic fatigue syndrome. But each month the malady upsets a woman's physical and emotional well-being. It can destroy personal and business relationships. It can be terribly self-destructive. And it can trigger such aggressive rage that in England and several other countries PMS has been used as a defense in criminal trials.

There are degrees of severity within each illness. Sometimes the illness goes into remission. At times it is progressive and leads to disability. At other times it is relatively mild. Occasionally it leads to diseases that cause death. Yet ICI, simply by being chronic, could be said to be severe. Illness that never ends cannot be taken lightly. As Mercutio said about his fatal wound in *Romeo and Juliet:*[13]

> 'Tis not so deep as a well, nor so wide as a church door, but 'tis enough, 'twill serve.

5

Being Chronically Ill

I know life could be worse. I could have only
one eye or leg, and I am very fortunate to have
all I do have . . . but those philosophies do not
solve the disease, do not get rid of the pain, the
tears, the frustrations, or the heartaches that
come with the problems.

Linda, a woman suffering with endometriosis

Diana, an adorable musician, reflects on chronic illness:

For the most part I have been proud of myself for how
well I have dealt with this illness. I have carried on with
my life without giving up. I've never stopped working
and I think I'm always there for my family. But during
this last attack, I felt so discouraged. I started looking
through the records I've kept and I realized that I began
not to feel well when I was twenty-five. I'm thirty-five
now, so that means that the last years of my twenties
and the early years of my thirties I have had to deal with
serious episodes of sickness and ten years of feeling pretty
lousy. I felt so sad. I know I haven't missed anything in
life because of being sick so often. I love my work and
my career has grown. I got married when I was thirty-
two and we're happy. But I guess I felt sad for myself—
sad for anyone—whose twenties and thirties have to be
shadowed by poor health. Maybe my forties and fifties
will be better. My life isn't in any way unbearable, but
every day when I wake up I have to confront my poor

body and transcend its pain and then get on with my day.

Most illnesses follow a typical process:

1. Warning signs of discomfort or onset of illness
2. The period of illness itself
3. Recuperation or convalescence after the illness
4. Recovery to health

Chronic invisible illnesses are different. They do not follow the predictable path from warning sign to recovery. Rather, the sufferer lives with a baseline of unwellness that is interrupted by periods of exacerbation and remission, relapse, and remission.

The person with ICI suffers a general sense of not feeling well and is challenged to adjust to that state and even to accept it. She must go about life with pain and discomfort, finding it difficult to achieve goals and projects, finding it hard to look her best, and finding it almost impossible to sparkle, to experience a zest for living and looking at peak levels. Whether the illness leads to a disabling condition or not, the chronicity of ICI sets it apart from conditions that can be cured, conditions that follow the onset-illness-recovery process.

Adjustment to this state of unwellness is a daily challenge. Franklin Shontz describes the psychological state associated with health as one that is characterized by a feeling of well-being, vitality, and vigorous pursuit of life goals. Conversely, sickness, as described by Shontz, "is characterized by feelings of helplessness, dependency, continuous discomfort, and narrowness of attention with a corresponding increase in a concern for somatic stimuli and constriction of goals."[1] The following chart lists the contrasting characteristics of states of health and of illness.

Characteristics of Health and Illness

Remission (Health)	Exacerbation (Illness)
Independent	Dependent
Able to pursue goals	Goals set aside
Energetic	Lacking energy and vitality
Freedom from intensity of symptoms	Symptoms increase in intensity
Sense of well-being (physically and psychologically)	Physical pain and discomfort affect psychological well-being
Mobile	Impaired mobility
Normal functioning of body	Body fails to function normally
Essential optimism	Essential pessimism
Able to control events over which control can ordinarily be exercised	Unable to have control over ordinary events
Able to fulfill such roles as mother, father, worker, lover	Not only unable to fulfill roles but unsure as to new role during illness
Little contact with the health-care world	Frequent contact with the world of health care—treatment, tests, medication
Able to give attention to others	Withdrawn from others to conserve inner resources
Personal focus can shift from self to others	Tendency to focus on self and somatic concerns
Able to contemplate the future with equanimity	Afraid of the future
Assertion	Passivity

The patient with ICI has known health, felt vigorous, and independently pursued goals and dreams. Then she must adjust daily to illness, sometimes severe, sometimes in remission, but the sense of health and vibrancy is never fully present and frequently it is diminished. Trudy, who has MS, describes the prospect of living with ICI,

Although most of the symptoms are not noticeable to most people, I never feel well. Imagine the sense of finality of never being able to bound out of bed in the morning saying, "I feel great!" There is not one small fraction of time when I am without a symptom of this disease.

Deirdre danced professionally for a dance company in New York after years of training. As a teen-ager she had followed her dream of being a ballerina, commuting daily into New York City for ballet lessons, practicing for hours with youthful energy and commitment. She was talented, won scholarships, and met high goals set by herself and her teachers. Her body was a finely tuned, disciplined instrument that responded to her will and vision.

Today, with CFIDS, Deirdre, even on her best days, is never unaware of the limits of her body. She tires from a flight of stairs. Daily plans must be designed around a low level of energy. She remains ambitious, but her activities are always restrained: teaching dance has been abandoned, her work must be sedentary, sports like golf and skiing are pursued but gently and with major restrictions. She adjusts. But she finds it painful to attend ballets. She reacts with awe and envy when she sees others pursuing simple daily activities—riding bikes, jogging, carrying children, mowing lawns. She does not know whether some day she will regain her strength and be well enough to teach dance again. When she looks toward her future, she is wary of making plans, not knowing whether she will be healthy enough to fulfill them.

Planning is a natural human activity. We plan our activities for the day: get up at seven, walk the dog, eat breakfast, be at work by nine, finish the work project, complete the deal, call our mother. We plan our families, our wardrobes, our vacations, our retirements. There are practical limits to our planning, like finances, but we enjoy the freedom of setting goals and meeting them.

For the sufferer of ICI, planning is problematic. A vacation set in April may have to be abandoned in June. Since airlines are not sympathetic, can one even make reservations? Should all life be put on hold? Projects as small as planting bulbs in the garden on time may be impossible to complete. Trying to plan a family may lead to despair. The planning that most of us do naturally, the patient of ICI does with an ominous sense of whistling in the dark. This inability to plan ahead severely limits personal enjoyment and achievement and greatly strains social life and relationships. "The family needs to know." "Can we or can't we?" This interpersonal strain is part of the difficulty in adjusting to the chronicity of the illness.

Adjustments to Exacerbations

As difficult as it is for the patient to adjust to and accept this constant state of unwellness, periods of exacerbation of the illness present an even more formidable challenge. When the disease attacks, unwellness shifts to almost unbearable sickness. Pain can be so severe as to make movement agonizing. Driving an automobile might be hazardous due to blinding headaches or blurred, double vision. Leaving the house can invite humiliating falls or shameful accidents. If the patient has doubted actually being ill, at times of exacerbation her agonizing handicap removes all doubt, but the doubt is replaced with excruciating, life-limiting pain, exhaustion, and a host of discomforting symptoms.

Ted described his experience of migraine attack as one might describe a nightmare:

> For nearly a year I had not had a headache. I began to think that they were really a "thing of the past." Then, a few weeks after we finished an addition on the house, I had a headache. It wasn't too bad. In fact, I just took a couple aspirin and it went away. Usually, when I have migraine headaches, they do not go away with aspirin. A few days later, in the middle of the night I started to

feel a migraine coming on. They have not stopped since. This has been about three weeks. All of a sudden I am back into this horrible world of pain. I feel like I can't stand, sit, or lie down. Sometimes I find myself just standing in the middle of the room. I want to tear my hair out or bang my head against the wall—anything— anything to get away from this constant pain. My children kind of steer clear of me during these times. I don't blame them, but I feel like a leper. They are frightened of me. So is my wife. Everything in our family comes to a standstill until the headaches are over. I feel guilty that we don't get things done and my wife wants to continue on as if nothing is wrong and make all the decisions. I can't help her because it's hard to think. I just have enough "mental" energy to get to work, do my job, and come home. Some life.

When the person is suffering from an exacerbation, which can last from a day or two to several years, his life is forced to change. Whatever changes he had made in his life to accommodate his illness now must be greatly adjusted. Projects that demand much physical energy usually have to be scrapped or postponed; plans that require great concentration are abandoned. Even shopping, caring for the baby, weekly tennis dates have to be curtailed or stopped. A woman who is afflicted with migraine headaches wrote to us after hearing us lecture:

I was glad to hear you include migraine headaches in your discussion of invisible chronic illnesses. We have two migraine people in our house, my daughter who is ten and myself. I was under tremendous pressure from my bookkeeping clients to do their year-end work and Shannon had four serious migraines. She lay balled up on the couch with the tears running down her face in pain so severe that she could no longer function. Unfortunately, when your own personal world stops, the rest of the world does not slow down and wait for you to catch up. The frustration—for her in falling behind in her school work and for me because as her world comes to a halt mine does also—is at times almost overwhelming. This same week I also had two migraines. It seems that we try to keep functioning into the migraine as long as we can and then finally reach a point where we are unable to function.

Since I am a single parent with no one to pick up the pieces, life unravels. If I'm the one with the migraine, basics like dinner just do not get accomplished and I become very unavailable to my child emotionally and physically.

As disappointing as it is to accept the limitations imposed by illness, worse still are the severe shame and embarrassment, as well as tension, that come in trying to communicate these limits to others.

Ann works on a team of four or five architects whose task it is to prepare proposals for a major urban construction company. On these projects, each team member plays a key role. And for each project there are tightly defined deadlines. When Ann is suffering a particularly severe exacerbation of endometriosis, she must drop from the team. Ann has prided herself on a lifelong attitude of "stiff-upper-lip, can-do, never complain." It is, therefore, very difficult for her to admit that she is unable to work. To communicate to the other team members—all men—why she is having to take time off is acutely embarrassing. In addition, she fears that they will view her as a female who can't bear pain or suggest that the reason women don't succeed in business is because they are too moody, too fragile, too subject to PMS. Ann fears that if they really knew the severity of her pain and the frequency of the attacks, they might remove her from the team and assign her to more clerical work.

Periods of exacerbation push the patient into the ranks of the truly handicapped. Standing in line in a store becomes unbearable, so articles are not bought or groceries are left in the shopping cart. Steps cannot be climbed, so many friends' homes, doctor's offices, and theaters are out of bounds. Some means of transportation are inaccessible. Before the exacerbation all these places and activities presented little or no problem at all. The patient has little time to adjust to being handicapped, and neither do friends, employers, and even bus drivers who have seen her normally going about life. Andrew describes an exacerbation of MS:

> I was driving home from work one day and I felt this numbness in my right leg. I didn't pay too much attention to it. I thought it was probably numb from driving. But the next day both of my legs were numb and then walking was strange. I would stumble a little. I have never really been sick in my life. I've had colds and things like that like everyone else gets, but I have never been seriously sick.
>
> I told my parents that I thought something was wrong and they encouraged me to see a doctor. By the time I did a week later it was pretty evident that I really had a problem. I couldn't walk without stumbling and the numbness was all the way up to my hips. I went into the hospital and I was there for about three weeks and was completely unable to walk. You can't imagine what it is like to suddenly become handicapped. I had to depend on someone to help me do everything, including going to the bathroom. My parents would come and see me every day and they looked so sad. They didn't know what to say to me, and frankly, I didn't feel like talking.
>
> I'm a lot better now. I can walk fine, but I don't know if it will happen again and I don't know if I'll ever be able to play sports again. Even though I can walk fine I tire easily. Sports have always been a big part of my life. Everything has changed and it's not easy to face it.

An added difficulty in adjusting to being handicapped with ICI is the phenomenon of appearing well. How paradoxically frustrating it is to fear the puzzled "But you look so well" when you feel disabled. Patricia, who has post-polio syndrome, reports that she is more and more frequently challenged by watchdog individuals for leaving her car in places reserved for the handicapped.

> I got a handicapped permit when I was having real difficulty with walking. I use it now when my legs aren't working well. But it gets so embarrassing sometimes. Yesterday, I was walking from the car and this guy came up to me and aggressively said, "Do you realize that parking place is for the handicapped?" When I said that I did and didn't he see my parking permit, he said, "Right, and I suppose you want me to believe that you are handicapped?" I wanted to cry. first because I was so embarrassed and secondly because I was so angry that I had to defend my right to park in the handicapped parking. I feel like I should carry a cane with me so I won't have to deal with people like him, but I resent that I have to prove my illness to anyone.

The periods of exacerbation are extremely difficult to endure, not only because of the pain and limitation, but also because of the fear that they engender. The patient lives in fear that the disease may seriously worsen, threatening not only his quality of life but even his life itself. And then, for no apparent reason, the disease attacks, sometimes in a totally new way. The ever-present fear is now felt in force. "Will I have to suffer this way for the rest of my life?" "Is this even the beginning of the end?" The fear and the unanswerable questions, together with the agonizing exacerbation itself, are almost unbearable. Clients tell us that at times like this that they often wish to die. Living with the pain or debilitating fatigue and the fear makes a final "simple" answer of death seem appealing. Rose, an artist who suffers from chronic fatigue syndrome, described her experience to us:

> I can't imagine a future with this fatigue. I'm not able to paint or to sculpt. I can't walk on the beach. I can't even enjoy the prospect of a visit with my grandchild,

whom I adore. I try to sew and continually have to let out the stitches and start over. That activity is about all that I can attempt at creativity. I find myself thinking of how I will kill myself and where and when. Then I think of the impact on my grandchild. I feel absolutely desperate.

Suicidal thoughts are frequent, terrifying companions of exacerbations. The despair stems from fatigue, from pain, from fear, from limits to one's lifestyle. But the hopelessness is connected also with the terrible ambiguity of ICI and the difficulty of coping with or adjusting to it.

The very nature of ICI and its unpredictable periods of attack and remission make any stage of coping that would lead to resolution beyond reach. When the person is in a low-level state of unwellness, accepting this state is very difficult in itself, but there is always the fear that the condition will suddenly and radically worsen. Then again, it might not, at least not for years. So what is the patient adjusting to: a poor but tolerable present, an unknown but potentially horrible future, or a future of ongoing low-level health? The disease sharply attacks any sense of health or well-being, which is agonizing to accept. It could worsen and totally ruin the patient's sense of life as worth living or it could gradually kill or it could leave next week as suddenly and unpredictably as it came. Attempting to adjust to that uncertainty is what can at times make death seem clear, simple, and desirable.

Adjustment to ICI
Remission

The victim of ICI is constantly adjusting activities, behaviors, attitudes, even her very sense of herself. When the disease is in remission of greater or lesser degree, the individual can feel rather healthy and "normal." Like those who are healthy, she experiences very few limitations, has little physical discomfort, is not dependent on others, and needs no contact with the medical world. Her self-image is active, independent, even vigorous and attractive.

Mona, a witty thirty-six-year-old real estate agent, described herself at those times:

> I feel like a part of the healthy, normal world. I do what I want to do when I want to do it. I feel pretty attractive. I begin to think that maybe I'm really not ill. I even feel a little phony about being considered sick. I know I've even limped away from my car with its handicapped license plates so as to look like I deserve it. Then boom! Two days later I can't go to church because I can't climb the steps.

When the illness is acute, the patient is back in doctors' offices, back in the hospital, back leaning on others, back feeling hopeless. Adjusting to such contrasting states can lead the person to feel as if she had a split personality.

Margaret is thirty years old. As the oldest of five children she has regarded herself as a responsible, nurturing woman. Now she is the mother of three—twin boys who are nine years old and a girl, Margy, who is six. Margaret loves to cook, keep the house immaculate, and be available always for Michael, her husband, and the children. Despite having lupus, Margaret has been able to fill these roles. But a recent exacerbation of her disease forced her to rest in bed to recuperate. In tears she described a morning during this period:

> It was unreal. I was lying in bed at seven in the morning instead of being in the kitchen preparing breakfast. I could hear the boys downstairs getting eggs out of the fridge and Michael telling them to be careful. Margy was offering to help. I couldn't stand it. Later I could hear Michael helping Margy get ready for school and then all of them leaving. I always see them off to school and check to see if they have books and lunches. I felt so helpless, like I wasn't even needed.

Lupus was forcing Margaret to experience herself in a new way. She was helpless rather than the always helpful mother. She was passive not active, lying down not bustling about. She felt worthless. Yet, neither Michael nor the children had ever seen her cry. She wanted still to appear strong and in command, but instead felt desperately weak and vulnerable.

Two months later Margaret was back on her feet. But Michael and the children, particularly the twins, had grown more self-reliant. They did much more for themselves. So as they were adjusting to her return as all-giving mommy, Margaret was trying to adjust to their new independence. Besides, she had grown somewhat used to Michael's caring for her, and now he stopped doing the little things for her that had made her feel loved: propping up her pillows, running the tub for her, bringing up her meals. She was adjusting to her old role as well as to Michael's. Even as she struggled to adjust, fear nagged at her that things would never be the same and that she was not the person she thought she was.

Living with the Exacerbation-Remission Phenomenon

Sickness can prompt, even demand, growth. Constant adjustment to states of health then illness, independence then dependence, confidence then doubt, strength then vulnerability, caregiver then patient tends to sap reserves of emotional well-being. There is no real point of resolution. The ICI sufferer cannot say once and for all, "All right, I'm sick, needy, dependent, and weak but with God's help I will accept what he has asked me to bear." She cannot become accustomed to being sick and dependent. When the exacerbation passes, the patient must adjust to a whole new way of being, feeling, acting, and thinking.

Adjustment to sickness is particularly difficult to one who, like Margaret, identifies herself and her self-worth with strength and independence. Sickness removes any sense of strength. When we are sick, we can't do what we formerly could do: work, play, achieve. We depend on others—and sometimes that condition has its rewards. Many of us have fond memories of being home from school when we were sick as children, allowed to lie in our parents' bed during the day, watch or listen to soap operas, and be administered to by mother with what Salinger called "consecrated cups of chicken soup." But more often being dependent is a humiliating experience to which adjustment is not at all easy. Having to be helped to the toilet, steadied as we walk, or spoon-fed can erase any sense of dignity. Submission to a doctor's authority, questions, scoldings, and treatment reduces us to the level of a naughty child. One psychologist who suffers from chronic fatigue immune dysfunction syndrome described a doctor's visit:

> I was kept waiting for forty-five minutes by a nurse who insisted on calling me "Mister" rather than "Doctor." Finally I was led to a small room and told to undress to my underwear. There I sat on the examining table—the only place to sit—without any reading material except diplomas on the wall for another twenty minutes. When the physician arrived without any apology at all for keeping me waiting and addressed me coolly as Mr.____, I felt furious. But like a schoolboy before the headmaster, I answered his questions. He ignored my observation that the fatigue and pain seemed more intense on hot and humid days and waved away a thought I had after reading an article in a medical journal regarding the disease. I'd love to have the arrogant ass in therapy, but instead I'm dependent on this guy who doesn't even listen.

As challenging as adjustment to sickness is, the adjustment to the ambiguity of ICI is even more demanding. Tolerance of ambiguity is a measure of patience and maturity, and like patience it might fit the adage: "Seldom in a woman, never in a man." The psychologist who above described his doctor's visit talked of the difficulty of adjusting to the uncertain. "If I know for sure what I have to deal with, then I can adjust to it. The same psychologist described this to be true in ordinary events:

Wednesday is my day off and, weather permitting, I play golf. If the weather is awful, I adjust to the fact and change plans. I go into New York for a matinee, or visit a museum or gallery. But if the weather is uncertain, then so am I. Should I go into New York? Should I go to the club and hope for the best? Should I wait for further news of the weather? I hate the ambiguity. My worst days off have been ones where uncertainty has kept me off balance and unsettled.

We want to know for sure so that we can come to terms with reality. Death of a loved one killed in battle is adjusted to more readily than having a son or daughter missing in action. How can we grieve, adjust, accept, unless we know what we are trying to accept? The victim of ICI struggles with this ambiguity. "What do I have? Is it mild or acute? When will it attack again? Will it get worse? I feel so well now—maybe I'm not really sick?" And just as sickness is most intolerable for people like Margaret for whom independence is self-worth, so ambiguity is most excruciating for those whose tolerance of ambiguity is low anyway.

Admitting Not Being Well

Someone suffering from invisible chronic illness follows a path from health to non-cure, a path strewn with baffling, disillusioning, discouraging obstacles. Symptoms do appear that threaten health, but they are often strange and therefore confusing.

Gina was excited to be having dinner at a beautiful restaurant in New York. She had settled into the plush banquet when she began to feel tired. She was a bit surprised since she had slept well the previous night and had not had a rough day. By the time the veal scallopini arrived she was drooped onto her date's shoulder and far too exhausted even to eat. A night's sleep had little effect on the fatigue, which persisted for about a week. The symptom was similar to natural fatigue but the usual remedy of sleep was ineffective. A few months later Gina had just arrived in Aspen for a week's skiing. The first evening began in the hot tub looking up at the mountain and sky while enjoying the combination of hot water and cool air. But out of the tub and starting to dress for dinner, Gina became nauseated and very tired. She toppled into bed, canceling dinner and a walk through Aspen. The following day she was well.

Again there were symptoms of unwellness—nausea and fatigue—but again seemingly without cause, rhyme, or reason. During the following months Gina would experience days of fatigue that seemed to sap her of all energy in a way that she had never previously experienced. Complaints drew puzzled responses from friends and family, but little sympathy and no help. Months passed and Gina began to have problems with her eyes; sometimes she would see double, and particularly at night her vision was impaired. Driving after dark became hazardous. She described her vision as clouded or seeing through a screen. It was the experience of the visual impairment that led Gina to the doctor.

Typically, people with ICI suffer from symptoms such as nausea, or headaches, or fatigue—all common ailments, generally caused by overeating or drinking or overwork or stress—for months before seeking medical help. These symptoms in healthy people are usually self-inflicted and self-treated, healed by rest, vacation, and over-the-counter medication. We make ourselves sick by too much fun or too much food or denial. We're responsible for getting ourselves ill and we're responsible for getting ourselves better. The victims of ICI are conditioned, like all of us, to feel responsible for being sick. Like all of us they search themselves for the cause of the malady (excess or omission of some kind) and attempt to get better. Their search leads, however, to confusion, self-doubt, vulnerability, and a sense of failure. It is in this weakened and helpless condition that they finally turn to the medical world.

Immediately there are doubts. "Who do you go to for fatigue? Are headache clinics worthwhile? Are any of these conditions connected? Am I causing them in some way? Am

I imagining them? Will the doctor think I'm crazy?" But the pain or the fatigue is awful, unbearable. So the conclusion is finally inescapable—go to a doctor and better start with the family doctor—"At least he'll be caring."

Arriving at this decision involves communication with family members and these interactions frequently intensify the patient's vulnerability. If Gina is viewed by parents or spouse as a complainer or as somewhat hypochondriacal, especially after weeks or months of complaining, their reactions to a proposed doctor's visit might be much less than sympathetic: "My God, you don't go to a doctor for fatigue, you stop working too hard," or "You're staying up too late," or "You've got to get it together and get going," or "You've never been too energetic," or "Gina, we all get tired—God, doctor's offices would be overrun if we all gave in."

Cost is also a factor. Because insurance deductibles are often very high, a doctor's visit is a very expensive choice. The patient accurately imagines that diagnosis of the myriad and confusing symptoms will probably entail several visits, extensive testing, and possibly referral to a specialist. Frequently, the patient puts off calling a doctor. She tells herself to put up with the pain or try another over-the-counter remedy or wait "till I can't stand it any longer." Besides, there is the constant underlying fear that all this is "in my head," that I might really be crazy. This fear is so terrifying that the thought of a doctor confirming the fear again results in choosing to "try to work it out myself."

Eventually, however, the suffering and doubt become unbearable and the person decides to call her doctor. By the time she makes the decision and visits the doctor's office, she is extremely vulnerable, self-doubting, confused, fearful, and needy. What she is about to experience often intensifies the worst of these feelings.

Violet, who suffers with severe CFIDS, was a pleasure to interview. She was open and informed and revealed an ascerbic sense of humor. She began the interview saying, "First of all I'm offended by the name chronic fatigue syndrome. We refer to it as chronic fatigue immune dysfunction syndrome (CFIDS)." She then went on to describe her harrowing years of inexplicable symptoms, search for a diagnosis, and treatment.

> I called myself a "mellow space case." I was a Transcendental Meditation teacher and a fitness instructor. So I thought I had learned to approach events in life with equanimity. One summer, my husband and I were traveling across the United States. It was a very good time in my life and I was really happy. Then symptoms began to surface. I had headaches, vertigo, adrenalin rushes, relentless fatigue, gastrointestinal problems, and memory loss. I went to so many doctors. I was Rolfed, acupunctured, cleansed, and put on vitamin regimens. I was told that I might have lupus. Another doctor told me that I could benefit from an assertiveness training program and another told me that my symptoms were signs of age.
>
> Finally, I was giving up on the system and I stopped going to doctors. I would only go if my husband "hit me over the head" and demanded that I try again. Then I learned of Dr. Paul Cheney and Dr. Daniel Peterson. I felt I was "led" to them and I joined many people who were searching for help who had read about these doctors' work.
>
> The day I was diagnosed with CFIDS, my husband and I went to the most expensive restaurant we could find, ordered dinner and a fine wine, and celebrated.

Violet is presently experiencing some relief from her symptoms with the experimental drug ampligen. She worries all the time that the drug will be removed from the market. But she had these words of advice for her fellow sufferers:

> You can come out of this. Some are luckier than most. We have to learn how to deal with this illness until a cure comes along. Keep in mind that each limitation opens new doors.

6

Seeking Answers,
Seeking Cures

> Be patient with all that is unresolved in your
>   heart,
> And try to love the questions themselves.
> Do not seek for the answers that cannot be
>   given,
> For you would not be able to live them,
> And the point is,
>   to live everything.
> Live the questions now,
> And perhaps, without knowing it,
> You will live along some distant day
> Into the answers.
>
> *Rainer Rilke*

The mind seeks truth and is not at all comfortable with the notion that there is no answer. For the ICI person and her family, discomfort hardly describes the desperate feeling of not knowing what the symptoms mean. They urgently need answers that the very nature of ICI defies. Unlike diseases such as diabetes or cancer, which have specific symptoms and specific treatments, the illnesses that we are discussing are usually diagnosed by a process of elimination, by ruling out other diseases. The patient, when first consulting a physician or later a specialist, complains of vague, varied symptoms. These complaints send the doctor off on a quest for diagnosis in any of many directions—blood tests, X-rays, CT scans. He usually finds nothing measurable to explain the pain, fatigue, or discomfort that the patient is describing. The doctor is persistent and tries more tests and further CT scans or MRIs. Eventually he concludes, for example, that due to signs of plaque on the brain the patient might have MS. The finding is not definitive; it is an educated guess or assumption.

Such a conclusion is deemed too terrifying for the patient, so many doctors would hesitate to state such a diagnosis. In his book, *Multiple Sclerosis: Something Can Be Done and You Can Do It,* Robert Soll suggests that in some instances doctors are reluctant to reveal

> a conclusive diagnosis because of their sense of the enormity of the disease. This well-intentioned attempt to protect the patient from bad news has just the opposite effect on an individual who has been living with curious and often frightening symptoms and is anxious for answers. More often than not, a patient suspects that there is something very wrong long before the physician tells him what it is.[1]

Faced with such equivocation, the patient then tries another doctor—and another—hoping to receive a diagnosis.

Evana, who complains of fatigue and periodic pain, is pursuing an insatiable quest for diagnosis. She admitted, when she came to see one of us,

> You're the third psychologist I've seen. I don't think I'm crazy but I don't have much hope that I'm ever going to find out what I have. So I figure maybe a psychologist can help me deal with it or figure out if maybe it's all psychosomatic. I have been feeling so sick for a long time. Some of my problems seemed like things my sister, who has lupus, complains of so I went to a doctor and took a number of blood tests. He says I don't have lupus. Then I read a book on hypoglycemia; I thought that was what I have because I feel so tired. I followed the diet the book suggested but nothing changed. Then a friend told me about a program she had seen on TV about chronic fatigue syndrome. I asked the doctor if I

could have chronic fatigue syndrome, but he wasn't too responsive. He said I have to be careful of fad illnesses.

The ICI patient suffers not only painful, often disconcerting symptoms but also agonizing restlessness. Is this symptom today caused by colitis or is it something else? Should I have it checked or just accept it? What if it's serious and could be treated? A tearful patient once called saying, "I honestly don't know if what I'm feeling right now is just in my head. I'm afraid that if I just tell myself to calm down and believe that the pain in my stomach is caused by my nervousness at going on job interviews, I will die of cancer because it wasn't detected in time. I hate the thought of bothering the doctor and I don't want him to think I'm one of those patients who is always crying wolf."

The search for knowledge is very much associated with a need for control. The unknown can be frightening and threatening. The cliché, "What he doesn't know can't hurt him," is not a comforting thought when applied to oneself. We want to know. Feelings that we cannot identify or explain are frightening. So is new pain. When we know the cause of the feeling or pain, the previously unknown becomes known, the unfamiliar is understood. We feel in control again.

The person with ICI suffers from a horrible sense of no control. He cannot control his illness—it has a course of its own. Exacerbations will come and go. He cannot control his fatigue or his pain. He cannot control his future by planning carefully. He can hardly plan next month's vacation because in his case surely "the best laid plans of mice and men gang aft aglee." Since such lack of control is very difficult to accept, the patient will attempt other forms of control.

For example, Howard, who has MS, lost the use of his legs. He became convinced that a new strict healthful diet, sleeping plan, and exercise regimen would someday help in recovering the use of his legs. He decided that his whole family could benefit from such a regimen. One morning he gathered his three children, wife, and mother together and proclaimed his plan for changes in the way they would eat, sleep, and exercise. Disallowing any opportunity for discussion, he insisted that they start with the new schedules immediately. Any disapproving comments from the children he countered with anger. His family regarded him as a tyrant. His approach was tyrannical, but his attempts to change his family's eating, sleeping, and exercise habits were a desperate effort to counter the circumstances that deprived him of the ability to support his family in a way that he believed "a man should." The attempt was a pathetic attempt to regain a sense of control.

Anne Marie, a thirty-two-year-old mother of two girls who feels no control over her chronic fatigue, lies in bed thinking, "I've got to get my files organized and the kitchen cabinets cleaned and straightened out and the clothes in my closet mended, cleaned, and pressed." Her planning would be beneficial if it were to preserve energy and avoid frustration. But for Anne Marie the intention stems from her need to have control somewhere in her life. Unfortunately, fretting over cleanliness contributes to restlessness and even to compulsive and exhausting behavior.

It is very difficult and very frightening for the patient of ICI to accept the reality that he has so little control over his illness. Even as he struggles to accept his lack of control, he hears of theories like those popularized by Norman Cousins, which propose that the way we think and live affects the course of our illness. These theories challenge him to change his way of being and to heal himself. The patient is told that he is responsible for his cure and guilty if he fails to achieve it. The message is clear: he can and must control his illness and himself.

Sandy first experienced the severe discomfort of irritable bowel syndrome when she was a teen-ager. Remarks made by her parents and a doctor about being more careful with her diet contributed to Sandy's feelings of responsibility for feeling sick. During her teen-age years and continuing into the present, Sandy, now in her thirties, has relentlessly pursued a cure. She has exhausted herself and exasperated those close to her in her desperate search. When we confronted her about the consequences for herself and her husband and family, she replied, "But there has to be a cure and I have to find it. What else can I do?" She has at last count been treated by at least twenty doctors, six chiropractors, one hypnotist, three masseurs, two dietitians, and an endless assortment of gurus practicing a variety of exotic healing techniques. Sandy's life revolves sadly and despairingly around her illness and her attempts to find a cure.

The ICI sufferer may be buffeted from two directions. First, he is the victim of skepticism and told that his illness is all in his mind. Then, when the illness is established, he may be victimized by theories that posit the mind as the all-powerful curative agent and challenge the patient to cure himself by good spirits. First he is the victim of materialists who doubt the illness because it cannot be measured, and then he is subjected to the demands of spiritualists who claim that he is responsible for the illness and its cure by his attitude and spiritual courage.

Responsibility for our health shapes the way we eat, rest, play, and exercise. To enjoy life in a healthy way we need to attend to our diet and to the condition of our body. Our mind, attitudes, and beliefs lead us to positive, life-affirming, peaceful ways of being that let us live at peace with ourselves and our world. But when that responsibility demands that we be accountable for our illness and for curing it, we become tyrants to ourselves.

Clients meditating for serenity, removing fat and sugar from diets, taking megadoses of vitamins, and pursuing gurus who promise cure-alls project a desperate need to be healed and to feel well. They are also manifesting other needs: for control, for understanding, and for hope. To become more peaceful and more accepting of the illness and of themselves, they need to recognize and respect these needs and to learn how to meet them.

If you suffer from ICI you need to learn to discriminate what you can control about your illness and about yourself and what you can't. In your frustration at not being able to control so much of the time so many of the physical symptoms of your illness, you can feel totally helpless and hopelessly out of control. But you are not. There is much you can control and much you need to control in order to live in as healthy and satisfying way as possible.

You can control yourself in more and more mature ways. You can increase control over your thoughts, disciplining your mind to focus on the present while avoiding the tyranny of "what if's" about the future. You can control your ways of relating with others, growing each day more honest with your feelings, more understanding of those around you, more controlled in your demands and complaints. You can develop more positive, realistic attitudes, and you can control negative, self-pitying ones. You can control imprudent behaviors and learn behaviors conducive to your health and well-being. You can control your tendency to think that you have no control.

You have a need to understand—and that need is understandable. While avoiding an endless search for the final curative answer, you can develop a keen and healthy interest in all that is known, however sketchy, about your illness. You can learn about possible steps to limit the virulence of its symptoms and what is best for you to do and to avoid. You can learn about the emotional as well as the physical characteristics of your illness and come to understand how your illness affects you physically.

You need to have hope. While avoiding unrealistic hopes that you are cured during periods of remission or overly optimistic reactions to publicized reports of scientific breakthroughs, you can hope for an increased capacity to cope with your illness. You can hope to learn new ways of accomplishing tasks despite fatigue and pain. You can hope to accept your illness more graciously. You can hope for patience and for growth in those qualities that make us more human, such as wisdom, courage, humility, generosity—qualities that often have adversity as their sources and root. And you can hope for continued growth in peaceful self-acceptance, self-appreciation, and self-knowledge.

Perhaps control, understanding, and hope can be fostered by responsible self-experimentation. You know yourself better than anyone else does. You can know yourself more by experimentation with what is and what is not beneficial for you. For example, consider exercise. You may find that certain exercises develop stamina and strength. Or you may learn that exercises reduce already low energy resources. Or you may find that the exercises appear to give both results depending on different circumstances. Eventually, some self-knowledge may result regarding when, how much, and what kind of exercise is beneficial. Such discovery might reduce feelings of helplessness and lead to feelings of greater self-acceptance. Even if the outcome is to find that exercise is virtually useless, if you arrive at this conclusion by yourself with personal experimentation, it might make the fact somewhat more acceptable.

A peaceful acceptance of self with an appreciation of one's gifts and one's limits is as rare as it is attractive. Self-dislike seems more common. Those who are obnoxious in their self-aggrandizement hide themselves from themselves. The individual who trusts himself, who knows his beliefs, his values, his needs, and his feelings is far better able to cope with whatever life has to offer—from praise to blame, tragedy to honors, sickness to health.

With this sense of self, the person afflicted with ICI will accept limitations without undue fear of being worthless, will say yes to an operation or no to more tests with relative calm and self-assurance. Without a sense of self-worth, the ICI patient is the frantic puppet of whichever doctor, guru, friend, or foe is pulling the strings. Meditation, diet, finding the best doctors—all are responsible behaviors that can enhance the quality of life. Frenzied search for a cure can destroy the patient, his life, and his relationships.

7

Consulting a Doctor

When you're cold don't expect sympathy from someone who's warm.

Aleksandr Solzhenitsyn

By the time a person suffering unknowingly from an invisible chronic illness decides to consult a physician, she has usually endured weeks or months of baffling symptoms. She has been alarmed by previously unknown sensations: tremors, sudden and complete exhaustion, pain that arrives without an observable cause and leaves just as mysteriously. She has feared that she has contracted a strange disease or that she is imagining things or that she is losing her mind. She has often driven family members from confusion to sympathy to skepticism to fear to impatience. She might have exhausted her listeners and been hurt and disappointed by their reactions. As she readies herself for her first doctor's appointment, she hopes for a complete and thorough response that will answer all of her questions and vindicate her with her skeptics. Yet, she fears that she will be met with more skepticism—professional this time, more humiliating and more confusing than any previously endured.

So the prospective patient tends to expect too much and too little. She also feels the pressure of friends and family who want either to help her or to have some answers to their doubts. The first visit can become an event surrounded by concern and questions:

"When do you go?"
"Do you want me to go with you?"

"Do you want me to be home tonight so that we can talk about it?"

"Did you write everything down?"

"Call me as soon as you leave his office."

"Will you go to work afterward?"

"Do you have the insurance card?"

"Did you take a check?"

"Do you have the directions?"

Burdened with family concerns and with her own hopes, fears, and expectations, the patient makes her first visit to a doctor concerning her ICI symptoms. After waiting uncomfortably and for what seems like an interminable stretch of time in the waiting room looking at magazines without absorbing any of the contents, she is led into another room and told that the doctor will be with her shortly. Now there are not even magazines to distract her. She sits, looks at walls papered with diplomas, and waits. The next words she hears will be the brain-stopping, "What seems to be the problem?"

The doctor asking that question comes to the patient with his own agenda. Physicians, by training if not also by aptitude, are scientific. They work with measurable phenomena. Blood pressure, temperature, brainwaves, and white blood cells can be gauged numerically. X-rays, EEGs, and MRIs can be examined and to the trained eye divulge information. Physicians, unfortunately, are not always endowed with the insight and patience to respond to the myriad, immeasurable symptoms usually endemic to ICI. Pain, though known to us all, is not really susceptible to measurement, and fatigue not only defies measurement but is so common as to be dismissed.

The patient is looking to be validated in her complaints, understood in her fear and confusion, respected in her ordeal with painful and mysterious symptoms. The doctor is looking to measure the data and to draw conclusions as to the possible ailment and its treatment. Medical school has trained his focus onto scientific examination of data—and the data that he too frequently ignores are the feelings and needs of the patient.

Miracles of medical technology invite the physician to further respect science. He is often poorly prepared to listen humbly and patiently to the confusing, inconsistent, non-measurable complaints of the ICI sufferer. Dr. Arthur Kleinman, author of *The Illness Narratives,* notes, "I recognized that my medical training systematically educated me about the former [medical issues] but tended to discount and in certain ways even blind me to the latter [life experiences of the person]."[1]

By the time of the first visit, the person with an ICI is so vulnerable and self-doubting that her reporting of the ailments is often sketchy and incomplete. Frequently, she withholds certain details due to embarrassment or fear that "If I told him that, he would surely think I was imagining it." When one adds the frequent sexual difference and prejudice between patient and doctor, the odds of full disclosure and understanding are poor. The patient of these diseases is often a woman; the doctor is often a man. Fear can inhibit the woman's full disclosure of her suffering. Most women are not conditioned to expect male understanding of "mysterious" female ailments. Male doctors too often disregard complaints of their wives or patients as typical female exaggerations.

The story of Mikko Mayeda, a blind equestrian who suffers with multiple sclerosis, dramatizes the crushing consequences to the patient of the physician's failure to give merit to the patient's complaints. When Ms. Mayeda was fifteen, she injured her knee in a sports accident. Surgery was necessary to repair the damage to her knee. While the surgery was successful, the once happy, active, straight-A student turned despondent. As Mikko tells her story, the surgery marked the beginning of a nightmare.

> I felt something was wrong with my body. None of the doctors would listen to me. They seemed obsessed with the idea that I didn't want to live. I did; I just knew

something was wrong. Well, they admitted me to a hospital where I was kept for nine months on medications. I couldn't call my family or friends and I couldn't have visitors for months. I was in a stupefied state. That's the way they kept me. I think that's the way they liked me.

Then I started to lose my coordination. My legs wouldn't work right. I tried to get someone to listen to me, but no one would so I gave up. What does a fifteen-year-old know? Those months in the hospital were horrible.

Finally, they let me go home. But I felt really out of it. I had been away from my friends for almost a year. I didn't fit in with my peers.

Life was very difficult the next couple of years and then I began to lose my sight. Again, no one would really listen to me or believe me. One day I was riding on my moped, it was late in the day and I was going about 30 mph. I hit something and crashed the moped. My face was crushed. When I was in the hospital a doctor examined my eyes and noticed optic nerve damage—pallor of the optic nerve. You know this is typical of MS. He suspected MS but didn't tell me. At that point the doctors suspected MS, but they wouldn't say it because there were "no other symptoms." Even though I had talked about how weird my body felt and about my loss of coordination.

That's when I really didn't want to live. Here I was twenty and going blind and I still didn't know why. Then my condition worsened. The disease affected my bladder and my legs. Eventually I was bedridden. Now I know I have MS, but the whole experience was terrifying and humiliating.

Mikko Mayeda's sad story of misdiagnosis is an extreme example of a common phenomenon in cases of ICI. Without hard data, the doctor often opts for a diagnosis of "hysteria" or "stress." Henri Baruk, author of *Patients Are People*

Like Us, notes, "Today when the physician cannot decipher a given set of symptoms and all the tests show negative results, he says that the problem is 'functional' or 'hysterical,' two formulas which cover a vast gulf of ignorance."[2] After hearing such complaints as numbness, fatigue, weakness, and headaches he will often ask, "What is your relationship like with your spouse?" "How long have you been divorced?" "Do you enjoy your job?" "Are you active?" These questions might provide the doctor with information pertinent to the patient's living condition that might be exacerbating her illness. But the vulnerable patient can get caught up in answering these questions and even begin doubting herself—"Maybe I'm really not happy or active or fulfilled in my marriage and if I'm not maybe that is why I don't feel well." She may realize only after leaving the doctor's office not only how humiliated she feels but also how frustrated that she was distracted from sharing some of the symptoms that she has been experiencing.

Other doctors will in half-listening or in impatience or in confusion make a guess followed by a prescription: "Try coffee in the morning for fatigue; try this pain killer; try getting more rest." Thus the scientist isn't even scientific; he doesn't pay rigorous attention to detail, investigate the symptoms more seriously, seek the advice of colleagues, or research his findings. Like others, the doctor becomes an impatient problem-solver.

Suzy's experience of her first doctor's visit is sadly typical.

> I waited, half-clothed, a long time for the doctor to come into the examining room, which made me feel vulnerable in the first place. But the doctor seemed pleasant and I was so anxious to find out what was happening to me that I focused on what I wanted to tell him. He asked me, "What is troubling you?" I began to tell him and he seemed to be listening, but he was examining me at the same time. He looked in my ears and eyes and he took my blood pressure you know, all the usual things that a

doctor does. At the end he said, "So, you feel like you are losing your balance?" When I said, yes, he said, "Why don't you walk down the hall for me," which I did. He remarked that my walk seemed pretty steady to him. I got flustered because I had tried to explain to him that it didn't happen all the time and that I wasn't surprised that I was walking fine. I felt embarrassed—like a kid caught in a lie.

But I still needed to know why I was occasionally losing my balance. When I pressed him on it, he didn't say that he didn't believe me, but at the same time he didn't ask me any more questions. He didn't suggest that I see a specialist. He just encouraged me to rest and said that if it happened again I should call him. I wanted to cry, but I was afraid that if I did it would just confirm for him that I "needed rest."

There I was, after all the time I took to decide to go to the doctor and all the anxiety I had gone through each time I lost my balance, still in the same position as I had been before the doctor visit. No wiser and a bill in hand. He seemed irritated with me when I persisted in asking questions.

Despite the often dissatisfying visit with the general practitioner, eventually, on his advice and also out of near despair with ailments, the patient reluctantly visits a specialist. If the general practitioner found it difficult to listen patiently to immeasurable symptoms, the specialist too often seems out of overwork or disinterest not to listen at all. Our clients tell of experiences all too similar and all too painful. Some specialists seem frequently to ignore the personal dimension of the doctor–patient relationship, often positioned above and beyond the patient and making no effort to relate warmly or caringly. These doctors dismiss the patient's thoughts, self-reflections, and feelings with an impatient tone. An American Hospital Association study revealed that the most common complaint of patients is that their doctors lacked compassion and failed to listen. Dr. Frankel of the University of Rochester Medical School, which conducted the study, said, "Patients would complain their physician never looked at them during the entire encounter, made them feel humiliated or used medical jargon that left them confused."[3]

Fear and distrust block self-disclosure. In the presence of non-care and non-listening the patient will often not reveal all that she is suffering. Many of our clients report being very selective in what they reveal to a physician. They know that their symptoms can be taken as signs of depression or neurosis and so they learn to avoid feeling language like "I'm frustrated (or discouraged or fearful)." They are aware that they can be quickly judged as depressive and forwarded to a psychiatrist.

Even when patients try to describe their symptoms, physicians are often not listening. Dr. Frankel, reporting on the American Hospital Association study, stated,

> The problem is that physicians too readily assume the patient's first complaint is the most important. But we find there's no relationship between the order in which patients bring up their concerns, and their medical significance. For most patients we've studied, when their physician gives them the chance to say everything on their mind, their third complaint on average is the most troubling.[4]

Dr. Frankel pointed out that the non-listening behaviors of physicians prevent patients from getting to their third complaint. In a study of the medical interviews between internists and their patients, fifty-one of the patients were interrupted within the first eighteen seconds of beginning to say what was wrong with them.

Some physicians try to substitute ersatz listening for genuine empathy. They say, "I understand," but they don't make the effort to listen deeply. Some offer grandfatherly care, "You must rest, dear," or "Why don't you take a nice long vacation—get a break and see new places." Some just give the problem-solving advice without the gentle tone.

True listening is very challenging. Sadly, some doctors listen even less than a helpful neighbor. Some doctors don't listen or relate meaningfully to protect themselves from the pain of seeing patients deteriorate, some out of their own feelings of inferiority and some because of a lack of interpersonal skills. It is crucial that doctors grow to know themselves and develop their ability to listen and to relate effectively.

The demand on the physician to listen is formidable. Within a brief segment of time, his task is to establish a diagnosis and prescribe a treatment designed to treat the malady as effectively as possible. To this end, he must listen for what is salient, sorting the essential from the irrelevant, deciphering what is symptomatic of illness from what is evidence of psychosomatic complaints.

A neurologist whom we respect summed up the daunting task he faces up to twenty times a day.

> I know that the patient wouldn't be in my office if he weren't suffering in some way. I am aware of how much this person needs me even if he's acting hostile or indifferent. I pray that I am attentive and caring even if I'm tired or irritable. But it's not easy. I have to leave the patient who is very annoying and immediately face another patient without carrying the annoyance with me. Or, I get off the phone with the hospital where some intern has screwed up the medication of a patient and not take my frustration out on my next patient. I feel terrible when I haven't been the way I would like to be with a patient. Other times I resent like mad the way the patients act—some of them are very hard to take.

The doctor must rely on the self-report of the patient while listening with an ear educated by training and experience. He has to enter into the world of the patient with skepticism kept at bay and empathy at the ready. "Entering into" the world of the patient through listening is all the more difficult since the doctor needs at the same time to "step back" to see the whole picture in order to diagnose the illness. If he steps back too far, he may remove himself from trusting contact with the patient and retreat into personal prejudice. Then judgment replaces trust:

"She's hysterical."
"He's narcissistic."
"He's a bore and a whiner."

Judgment replaces respectful attention or careful, professional diagnosis. The doctor needs to be aware of his personal prejudices. The patient needs to be aware of the challenge facing the doctor. Each has responsibilities in the creation of a trusting, beneficial relationship.

The doctors who master their daunting and sacred task are the ones who listen most skillfully and profoundly. They demonstrate genuine concern and compassion and admit the limits of their knowledge. These professionals are as deeply comforting as their non-listening colleagues are depressing. The issue of how patients and doctors need one another and how they need to relate will be taken up in chapter 15.

From his experience in seeing many patients, a doctor is in a unique position to understand and to relieve the self-doubt and shame of the patient. Stephanie, who suffers from chronic fatigue, described her response to her doctor:

> I had just about given up hope that I could get help. I had been to four doctors over the last three years and each time came away feeling foolish or humiliated. Then I heard about this woman neurologist in Connecticut. When I first met her, I was taken aback by how young and pretty she looked. Then I couldn't believe how she let me talk, how she seemed to respect my experiences of fatigue as valid ones. In fact, she seemed to know just what I was talking about. She hasn't promised a cure, but she has said there are things that we can try. Maybe there's hope. At least there's someone with experience who takes me seriously.

A doctor can and should be a source of support, comfort, knowledge, and healing. Unfortunately, for the ICI patient, he is too often a source of distress. In Chapter 15 we will discuss ways that you can help the medical profession to help you. There are doctors who truly heal. It is your job to find them and to meet them maturely and effectively.

8

Relating with Family, Friends, and Colleagues

It is difficult to stand forth in one's growing, if
one is not permitted to live through the stages
of one's unripeness, clumsiness, unreadiness, as
well as one's grace and aptitude. Love provides
a continuous environment for the revelation of
one's self, so that one can yield to life without
fear and embarrassment. This is why love is in
the strictest sense necessary. It must be present
in order for life to happen freely. It is the other
face of freedom.

Mary Carolyn Richards

Where need is most pronounced, feelings are most
intense. In the loneliness of pain and sickness, we need
the comfort of care, sympathy, and understanding. We want
this comfort from those who know us best—our spouses,
family, and friends. When we are met instead with impatience and distrust, we are shattered. We withdraw like
wounded animals. Or we attack those who are hurting us.
Spouses and family members of the sick are often overwhelmed by their own needs and feelings. Their needs for
intimacy, companionship, and happiness are threatened by
complaints of sickness. Their feelings of fear, disappointment, confusion, hurt, and anger are complicated by feelings of guilt for being well and for having needs that the
loved one is often not able to meet.

Clashing needs and perceptions frequently lead to painful
conflict between the person with ICI and his family and
friends. To family and friends the patient often looks "just

fine." Often, even in the worst exacerbations, the illness is as we have named it—invisible. As the patient herself can be in doubt as to the realness of the illness, so can the ones who love her most. In addition, family members, like the sufferers themselves, practice denial. They would often prefer to think that the problem is psychological rather than admit that their daughter, son, or spouse has a major illness. Somehow a psychological problem may be resolvable. Their need is for her to be well; their perceptions or misperceptions are frequently shaped by that need. Such needs and perceptions can lead to behaviors that are annoying to the patient.

Linda is an art consultant for advertising firms. Her work requires that she travel from time to time. For the past six months she has had chronic pain in her neck, shoulders, and back. Her doctor believes that she is suffering from fibromyalgia, which can, he warns, be exacerbated by stress. Two years ago, after a divorce, Linda and her two-year-old son, Gregg, moved in with her mother. On several occasions Linda's mother observed Linda and Gregg's tearful goodbyes before Linda's business trips. Now she is convinced that Linda's pain is a result of their separation and remarks, "Do you think maybe you shouldn't go on this trip?" Then she advises directly, "You know, until Gregg is in college, wouldn't it be better to stop consulting work out of town?"

These unhelpful, misguided hints do contain a particle of truth. Linda does experience stress leaving Gregg. But Linda receives no empathy from her mother for the suffering that she is enduring at this moment. Her need for understanding is not met by her mother. In addition, she is annoyed by the advice and even thrown back into self-doubt—"Maybe it is, just stress after all," or "Maybe stress causes the exacerbation." The relationship with her mother becomes confusing and annoying, resulting in a tendency for Linda to avoid contact with her mother, which causes hurt on one side, guilt on the other, and more tension all around.

Regina also suffers from fibromyalgia. Frequently, her pain is so severe that she cannot work. Yet Regina has always found it difficult to say no to anyone. Even though she has been forced to resign from her job, she will still say yes to doing an errand for her father and brothers. Her husband is hurt and confused seeing this, since her not working has severely stretched their finances. With him she feels freer to be honest and to say no when he suggests visiting his parents or taking a weekend camping trip. Regina's difficulty in admitting her illness to others or in saying no to requests and invitations creates suspicion and anger in her husband, who thinks that only he endures her complaints and rejections.

People with ICI need to be trusted especially by those closest to them. But it is difficult to trust another person. We want evidence. If our child says he is sick on a school day, we look for outward signs of illness: a temperature or some coughing or vomiting. If someone asks for a donation, we want proof that the cause is worthwhile. When people say that they love us, we think, like Liza in *My Fair Lady*, "Don't talk of love, show me."

Appearances belie ICI. Despite looking "fine," the patient may be suffering greatly. Someone needing her to play, to make love, to work, to contribute has to trust that, despite appearances, she is not able. Such trust is difficult when one's perceptions have to be discounted; it is even more difficult when one's needs have to be denied. Disappointment, hurt, and anger strain the quality of trust. Realizing that she is going to be misunderstood or that behaviors might be expected that she cannot perform, the patient may tend to exaggerate her symptoms around those she loves. For example, if she is suffering fatigue, she might slump her shoulders or walk very slowly or talk in a tired, strained way. For these efforts she might be rewarded with lowered expectations, but more often her behaviors will be met with impatience and even distrust: "You don't have to act like you're dying!" or "Come on, let's speed it up." The patient again finds herself caught between contradictory wishes: wanting clear, convincing outward signs of her illness, yet praying desperately that the disease will not get worse.

Family members and friends of the person with ICI have their own conflicting wishes and needs. They want their spouse, daughter, friend to be able to work or play but they also need to be confident that she is taking care of herself. If they see her dancing, for example, they can be caught between feelings of joy, concern, or even irritation. Liam described to us his feelings regarding his wife, who has MS.

> I really don't want to nag her. She hates it and I hate it. But let me give you an example of how hard it is to refrain from nagging. I came home from work one day and she was coming into the house from the backyard. She was so happy to tell me that she had spent the day planting a lot of the seeds for the garden. I couldn't believe it. I wanted to yell at her that she was crazy to do so much work and in the hot sun. I knew she'd be sick and tired the next day when we were supposed to go out to dinner. I held back from yelling because she looked so happy. But she knew I was tense.

Just as mutual needs met create a solid base of satisfaction between people, needs not met on both sides tear away at the fabric of a relationship. Joan needs Bob's warmth, patience, and understanding. Bob needs Joan's sexual interest and vitality. Her endometriosis makes intercourse very painful. Suspicious and frustrated, Bob is in no mood to be warm and sympathetic. The issue does not remain simple: pain therefore no sex. Judgments born of hurt and anger rip at trust and understanding: "Now she has a new excuse—she's always been frigid." "He doesn't give a damn about me—he just wants sex."

Sometimes, MS causes impotency in men. Tom's wife related in therapy that he had demonstrated impotence previously in their marriage and concluded, "I think he's using MS as an excuse." Dennis's family is very active and has a tradition of an annual vacation where brothers, sisters, and their spouses come together for a week of sailing, golf, and tennis. Jane, his wife, has irritable bowel syndrome. She cannot predict when it will flare up. For summers she has agonized at these affairs, fearing shame and embarrassment, particularly when sailing. She feels like a blight on the scene. Recently, she has decided not to attend the annual gathering. Dennis's response, fueled by frustrated needs, was predictable, "You've never enjoyed my family. And you always seem well enough to go shopping with your sister. It's bullshit and you know it."

Jane is partly responsible for Dennis's judgmental reaction. Like many sufferers of invisible illness, she has denied or doubted her condition. Distrusting herself, she has at one moment pushed herself to appear totally normal and well and at another given in to a round of diets, doctors, and holistic medicine practitioners. Her lack of clarity and self-respect has matched Dennis's denial of his feelings and allowed him to dominate her with the forcefulness of false confidence and certainty.

Many patients doubt themselves and their disease. At times they do ignore signals from their bodies, push themselves, test their endurance. "Maybe if I just forget about it and walk normally. . . ." At other times, they feel that they will go mad attending to another symptom. Their own self-doubt and confusion are reinforced by those around them. There is always a sense of being distrusted: "Maybe if you tried harder." "Maybe if you rested more." "What if you see a psychologist—or a different one." "Well, what did the doctor say exactly?" In self-doubt and confusion, the patient is terribly vulnerable to the suspicions and misperceptions of those who should know her best.

The self-doubt and subsequent constant self-questioning are at the heart of the patient's torment. When Kim, who suffers from chronic fatigue, feels a wave of intense fatigue, the questioning begins: "Should I give up my job and find a more sedentary one? Did I bring this state on by not stopping chores and errands soon enough? Am I like this because I ate too many foods with sugar or because I stayed up too late? Am I responsible? Should I seek relief? Am I getting dependent on medication? Will the doctor get fed up seeing me again saying I'm tired?"

In this vulnerable state the patient becomes overly sensitive. A friend's simple question, "How are you?" is not simple for the sufferer of invisible chronic illness, who may be preoccupied with her body and with pain. To respond "fine" sets off feelings of resentment and loneliness; yet to talk again of pain or fatigue triggers fear of the other's impatience or rejection. A casual remark by a spouse that the kitchen cabinets are dirty or that there are spots on the rug can unleash a torrent of self-defense that is full of blame and self-pity. It is not easy to have ICI and it is not easy to relate intimately with the one who does. Later, in Chapter 16, we will focus on how to cope with ICI within the family.

II

Coping with Invisible Chronic Illness

> It doesn't matter what happens to you
> in life, it only matters how you cope
> with it.
>
> Rose Kennedy

9

Living in the Present

Each second we live is a new and unique
moment of the universe, a moment that never
was before and never will be again.

Pablo Casals

One of the greatest challenges for the person suffering with ICI is to live in the present moment, to keep her focus on today. Today might be immediately painful, might tax her limits of endurance, but she can cope if she does not allow an imagined future to add its weight to her burden and overwhelm her. Bernice describes a typical imagining of the future, an activity that for her usually provokes despair.

> I can't think of anything more unbearable than having a colostomy. Sometimes I dream and I get these pictures in my head. I get attracted to this guy, fall in love, get married, make love. Then the picture goes black and I get this attack of panic inside me. What if there is no further treatment for me and the only thing they can do is a colostomy? The thought sends me into despair and makes me feel hopeless about having a relationship. Maybe someone else could understand, but I can't envision asking someone.

We all have the natural tendency to think about our future. The tendency allows us to dream, to hope, to plan. "I'll have children, I'll get a graduate degree, I'll move to Colorado and live near the mountains." The natural proclivity to think about the future is necessary in making decisions. We project outcomes and consequences—a necessary part of decision-making. For example, if I choose Job A, I will get more money but probably less job satisfaction. If I choose Job B, I will have less money but I will enjoy the work more. We naturally try to imagine the consequences of each option and to choose the most desirable one. The trouble starts when we distort the natural tendency, when fear and pain trigger tyrannizing "what if's." Then our focus is on a future that terrifies us and leaves us helpless—a future for which no immediate plans or actions are required or even possible.

"What if I feel pain?" "What if I'm always too tired to work or to exercise?" "What if I lose the use of my hands or legs?" These "what if" imaginings render us hopeless and helpless. They have to be dismissed or challenged. Do they point to a concern for which we can take action? For instance, does "What if I'm too tired ever to go back to work?" point to a concern for which we can take action? Obviously not, so the question has to be banished as bogus and anxiety-producing. "What if I always feel pain?" No. As difficult as it might seem, we must get rid of the thought. It must go. What about, "What if I lose the use of my legs?" Nothing can or need be done about that today. So the question has to be dismissed from the mind.

Clearing the mind of futile, troubling thoughts demands commitment and concentration. Our fears produce these troubling thoughts quickly, push them to the front of our minds, and insist that we pay them close attention. Our anxious minds respond and grip the thoughts with addict-like force. We go over them and over them, as though we will obtain relief and arrive at answers. We do not. But we won't let go of them and we will not be able to without great effort.

If you are addicted to such thoughts, you need, first of all, to admit that they do you no good; in fact, they destroy serenity. Second, you must learn to recognize the thoughts as soon as they appear. Third, you need to learn how to drive them out of your mind before they do that to you. Sometimes even by making beeping sounds, out loud if need be, you can block their access to you. Sometimes thinking funny, happy, or peaceful thoughts pushes the anxious ones away. Sometimes turning your attention to some task that demands present attention works. Many of our clients have told us that they have been amazed at how the beeping sounds have been effective in routing the thoughts. The beeping can trigger one's sense of humor, which is anathema to anxiety.

No one can know for certain what his future will be like. In general, if we are feeling pretty well and have a healthy mind set, we don't worry much about the future. It is natural for us to spend some time and energy on future concerns and events. We need to look ahead, to plan, to anticipate. We save for rainy days, we plan for our children's education and for our retirement, we anticipate our vacations. Often looking forward to a holiday is half the fun. Nervousness before a big event is natural. It is equally natural, however, to reserve the bulk of our energy for coping with the task at hand and for enjoying the present experience. We have the resources to cope with present conditions and their limitations; we are helpless to deal with anxiously imagined futures.

Distortion of the balance between planning and enjoying right now occurs when anxiety and pain distract our attention so that inordinate amounts of time are spent worrying about the future. Other signs of this imbalance are visible when time and energy are used inefficiently, not in helpful decision-making but in paralyzing "what if's." These signs are also visible when existing needs and desires, such as those for rest, peace, concentration on a task, contact with others, enjoyment of daily pleasures, are given short shrift.

The person suffering with ICI needs all the peace and enjoyment that the present moment might provide. Sadly and ironically, it is the one who is anxiously suffering who tends to eye the future, the very one least likely to have a realistic view of it. Suffering tends to provoke anxiety, which in turn leads to projection of an anxiety-producing future.

Many ICI victims struggle to overcome this self-defeating tendency. Rita, who has MS, fights a rather typical inner battle:

> I hate waking up at night 'cause that's when I can't control my head. I start picturing myself bed-ridden. Jack [her husband] would wait on me, bring my meals up and stuff, but I know he's fed up already with me—I think that would tip him over the edge. How could I raise the kids? Then I think maybe he'd get custody. Then how would I survive? But why keep on anyway with Jack gone and no kids and no money? I lie there with these thoughts going over and over. I try to turn off my brain, but I can't.

Rita's suffering and anxiety have created a nightmare over which she feels helpless.

When we are thinking in this manner, we cannot remember that in the past we have suffered, imagined the worst, and then recovered. We forget that our imagined horrors did not happen. We don't learn from the past; anxiety brings on again the self-defeating, tortuous mind games. We even convince ourselves that such thinking is being honest—facing the facts. We don't realize that our imaginings are not facts at all, but terrifying, anxiety-producing, depressing creations of suffering and fear. They do not describe present reality or prepare us for the future. A frequently repeated, "What if I become crippled?" doesn't lead to a purchase of crutches or abandonment of a three-story house. And, "What if I go blind?" doesn't lead to classes in braille. These useless thoughts lead to nothing but anxiety and depression and sometimes to self-pity. Careful preparation for the future requires more rational thinking.

Irene, suffering intensely in the present from endometriosis, has been advised to have a hysterectomy. If she projects a lifetime of the pain that she is presently suffering, then she will do anything to prevent such an unendurable life from happening and might choose the operation. Her extreme pain prevents her from reflecting rationally about her life and goals. She is twenty-five years old. She has a loving fiance and both of them want a family. A hysterectomy might be a remedy, but it would also shatter her hopes of bearing children. She needs to balance physical pain with life goals. Such reflection is not possible if the brain is functioning only in panic fashion.

Some clients pride themselves on avoiding "what if" thinking about the future, only to find themselves involved in more subtle, even insidious forms of future thinking. Martha, who is sixty-five and has post-polio syndrome, says:

> I felt kind of proud of myself that I wasn't thinking, "What if I lose the use of my legs?" or "What if I have to quit my job?" all the time the way I used to. Then I caught myself just taking for granted that I would always have pain and it was subtly affecting the way I was making decisions and plans. I don't really know that I will always have pain, but I began to realize that a new kind of projecting into the future was going on inside of me without my being aware of it.

Living in the present makes sense, but it isn't easy. Carly Simon years ago sang about the cost of "anticipation"—thinking about what she would say on a date, about "How right the night might be." It is easy to fall into the belief that "thinking makes it so." It is challenging to enjoy the present moment without missing it to plan the next one. We look forward to a concert and fail to enjoy the drive with a friend or spouse to the concert hall. We might miss the pleasure of the music thinking about how late we will be going to bed, and how difficult it will be to get up, and how tired we will be at work. We miss the pleasure and nourishment of the present moment worrying about a time that is not present.

When the present is painful, fearing the future is hard to resist. Mabel, a sweet woman, confined to a wheelchair, moaned as she tried to wrench her mind away from terrifying thoughts of total dependence in the future.

> You say I should just stay in the present. The present is awful. My legs don't work, I'm worried about money, and I'm afraid disability won't cover my costs. I really try, you know I do. But sometimes I'd rather die than wake up and face all of this again. Then I start worrying about the future. I've been afraid of the future all my life. I always knew something was wrong with my legs but it took fifteen years and many, many doctors before I was diagnosed. Look at me now.

Living in the present is particularly challenging for ICI sufferers. The baffling, anxiety-provoking nature of the diseases as well as the progressive and exacerbating/remitting nature of some of them threaten living in the present. But such threats make living one day at a time all the more necessary for mental health and serenity. Elizabeth describes the process she went through to successfully resist focusing on the future:

> I had been in the hospital for the second time. At the beginning of the week, I was terribly sick and in pain. We—the doctors and my parents and I—were afraid that lupus had affected my kidneys, and we decided that I'd better be in the hospital so they could keep a watch on my condition. It turned out to be a false alarm—well, I should say, at least this time there doesn't appear to be any permanent damage. But, I'll tell you, that was when I began to think that I had to find a way to enjoy the times I feel healthy. I had gotten a glimpse of what it would mean to be so sick that I needed someone to help me get to the bathroom or wash myself. I don't feel well most of the time, but I can do those things for myself now. I realize, too, that I can do a lot even though so

many things are limited to me because I feel so tired
most of the time. I'm learning, day by day, to take pleasure in everything that I do. It's hard. Fear is always
there to start me worrying about what I'll be like next
year or the following one. Then I think of the hospital
stay and I force myself to focus on today. I hope other
people can do it without having an emergency or a hospital stay. It's a hell of a way to learn that to appreciate
the present is a much better way to live.

The challenges that we are discussing are all characterized
by periods of exacerbation and remission. Unless the ICI
patient is living in the present, during an exacerbation he
will project a lifetime of agony into the future. When he is
in a period of remission, he will either not enjoy the relief
due to fear that it will not last or he will project the relief
into a sense that the disease has gone away, even that it might
never have been real. The next exacerbation can then be
terribly crushing.

We invite you to become more conscious of enjoying the
present moment. That moment might be a conversation with
a friend, a restful bath, or a good meal. Letting the present
moment be truly nourishing might mean that you drink in
the beauty of a fresh morning, that you stop to listen to
your child's description of an event at school, that you listen
to the music that is playing on the radio rather than let it
fade into a musical wallpaper.

One client, in working at becoming more aware of the
present moment, described his experience of jogging:

> I have jogged every morning for years. Only recently
> have I begun to be aware of the satisfaction of my legs
> and arms pumping away. I feel the cool air on my face.
> I look at the trees against the sky. I feel my breathing
> through my chest and abdomen. I love it. Like I'm really
> into what I'm doing. Sometimes I will catch myself
> thinking about work, or about something I'm going to
> do. One time I had even stopped running I was so lost

in thought. Not that I consciously decided to. I had begun
to think of something else. I'm trying now to be very
present to running. Then maybe I can be more present
to wherever I am or whatever I am doing.

When we are present to our spouse, our friend, our work,
our prayer, we give ourselves to the person or activity and
the person or thing gives more deeply back to us. We draw
from a deeper part of our spouse or child or activity to be
more deeply nourished than we could ever be by the surface
only. A psychologist told us, "When I am really present to
my client, I hear more and see more. I feel energized and
time flies. When I'm distracted, not quite there, I feel tired
and the clock seems to crawl." Living in the present means
being aware, aware of my feelings, my needs, aware of who
and what is present to me at that moment. Remember a
variation of the Biblical saying, "Sufficient for the day is the
challenge thereof." It means controlling the mind from
creating a hopeless future. It means accepting the suffering
of today with grace and dignity, wisely realizing that today
is the only day I am responsible for living. I might be without pain tomorrow. I might be dead tomorrow. I will face
tomorrow when it arrives as today.

10

Thinking Clearly

Do not distress yourself with imaginings.
Many fears are born of fatigue and loneliness.

From the Desiderata, author unknown

The way we think governs the way we feel, which governs the way we behave. The conviction that our thoughts play an essential role in our lives is the basic premise of cognitive psychology. For example, if a person believes that he will be fired from his job for merely taking one sick day, he will feel fearful or angry in anticipation of telling his employer of his plans. His feelings may prompt him to put off informing his employer until the last minute, thereby risking a more negative outcome. Similarly, if a woman thinks that her fiance will call off their wedding when he learns that she has just been diagnosed with Crohn's disease, she will dread telling him. This feeling may prompt her to cancel the wedding herself. She will think that she is acting on logical self-protective grounds: "I'll reject him before he can reject me." She may live to pay a terrible price for her impulsive logic.

If our thinking were rational and conformed to reality, then our feelings would be justified and our behavior congruent with the facts. Unfortunately, our thoughts are very often irrational and reactive and these thoughts often go unchallenged. Cognitive psychologists call such thoughts "automatic." "If she criticizes my work, I'm no good, worthless, and could easily be fired." "If they don't like me, I'm a failure." When a shy person fails to speak up at a meeting, he might think automatically, "If I say anything,

I'll sound stupid." When a lonely man refuses to talk to an attractive woman at a party, he may be thinking, "She'd never want to talk to me." These automatic thoughts come to us like knee-jerk reflexes. They are immediate, involuntary, and irrational. Left unexamined and unchallenged, such automatic thoughts will trigger both anxiety and unproductive behaviors.

People with invisible chronic illnesses are prone to such anxious, self-defeating ways of thinking. John suffers from Crohn's disease. His thinking while contemplating surgery is automatic, irrational, and fatalistic. His anger and fear are very understandable, but his unchallenged thinking leads to self-pity and despair.

> I did everything that I was advised to do by my doctor. I really changed the way I ate and I tried to have as little stress in my life as possible. I took the medication religiously—I never missed a day. I thought if I did everything right, I wouldn't have to have surgery. I can't believe this is happening. I don't think I can survive this. I just don't have the strength after all I've lived through these past few years. This is unbearable.

John has fallen into automatic thinking that takes as true the belief that the situation is literally unbearable.

A person who believes that her self-worth is based upon her vigorous and effervescent way of being will function on that belief. Unaware, she may live by rules such as, "People won't like me unless I'm the life of the party," or "No one will ever go out with me unless I stay in shape." These thoughts rarely come into full consciousness, but they wield awesome power. Not only will this woman experience the physical exigencies of illness, but the contrast of illness to her typical way of thinking will threaten her sense of self-worth. She will make decisions based on these beliefs: "People won't want to be with me unless I can make them laugh and feel happy—I don't feel well and I don't feel bubbly and vigorous, so I can't make others happy, so, I won't go to the party tonight." It would be tempting to argue with her, "Don't worry. Come to the party and just be there. We'll be happy just to have you there." Unless she has brought her unreasonable beliefs into awareness, such encouragement would be futile.

These automatic thoughts are rooted in an underlying schema, that is, an unconscious organizing system about self formed early in life and confirmed through life experience. Imagine, for example, a child who learns very early in life that "being brave" is applauded in his family. The first time he goes to the doctor for vaccinations, his mother, the nurse, and the doctor all affirm him for not crying. The doctor remarks, "Now there's a good boy. You didn't cry at all." The nurse murmurs, "You were sure better than the little boy before you. He screamed at the doctor." His mother pats him on the head, saying, "I can always depend on you to be brave." The little boy ingests the notion that not demonstrating fear or hurt is the best way to act. So he goes off to camp without a word about his fears or he quietly endures his disappointment at being cut from the Babe Ruth baseball team. He develops an image of himself that is founded on the belief that "bravery" is the fundamental manner with which to approach events and people. He may unconsciously construe this belief to mean that he should keep his feelings of hurt and fear to himself. Such a goal easily leads to denying feelings even to oneself.

Now imagine this young man's attitude and behavior if he were struck with multiple sclerosis. The disease not only would exact its physical toll but would also threaten the very constructs upon which he has built his identity. He might decide, "I'll face this disease head on. No one will catch me feeling sorry for myself or giving into this illness." He may not consciously add, "This is the way I have dealt with everything in life and this is the only way that people accept me," but he surely will be operating on this conviction. He is then confronted with the characteristics of invisible illness. How does he bravely face an illness that at first he is not positive he has? How does he resist or ignore symptoms that are vague, baffling, and transient?

The schema that suggests that the only appropriate way to face life is with a commitment to demonstrate bravery at all times is faulty and rigid and fosters the belief that success in life and acceptance from others will be contingent upon the demonstration of courage. In our example, the young man may believe that if he doesn't face MS with silence and fortitude, he will let others down and will not be loved. His conclusions and decisions will lead to great dissatisfaction in relationships, depression in response to the ambiguity of the symptoms, and frustration at the lack of affirmation that he receives for "being brave."

Bringing faulty automatic thoughts into consciousness is central to successful and satisfying adjustment to the stresses of ICI. If we know the source of thinking that colors our perceptions, governs our feelings, and guides our behavior, we can experience a sense of control over ourselves—the very sense of control that invisible illness threatens. Only then are we able to stop saying, "This disease is controlling my life."

Not only does the patient have to learn to heighten awareness to automatic fallacious thoughts but so do those around her. Diana and her mother came to us several months after Diana had been diagnosed with endometriosis. Diana had come for several sessions by herself before she came with her mother. During these sessions, she had been open and sweet. As she sat across from her mother, however, she looked hard. She stared at her mother as if she faced an enemy, and she refused to talk. Her mother looked helpless and began talking with tears in her eyes.

> Diana was always the moody one of my five girls. Actually, she wasn't moody when they were all little girls. She was so active and lively. All five of them were adorable. My husband would always brag about his lit-tle women. People would stop and look at them when

they were all dressed up. But, oh dear, when Diana became a teen-ager, did things change. She was really unbearable sometimes. I used to wonder and wonder, "What did I do wrong? What could I have done better so she wouldn't be this way?"

Diana's mother was unable to accept Diana's illness. In therapy she became more aware that her inability to face Diana's illness was founded on the belief, "I am a good mother if all my daughters are healthy and happy." Thus, she perceived Diana's complaints of pain and fatigue as reflections of her failure. Therefore, each time Diana cried in pain or stayed in bed, her mother chastised her. Diana was furious with her mother. She resented that her complaints were never met with sympathy but always with impatience and disbelief. Mother and daughter became enemies instead of companions in search of ways to ease Diana's pain. Embroiled in such conflict with so important a person in her life, Diana had difficulty coming to terms with her illness. Her energy and her mother's were dissipated in acting out automatic thoughts and destructive judgments.

Automatic thoughts prevent awareness of feelings, needs, and expectations and lead instead to "programmed," ineffective action. For example, a businessman, Andrew, who struggles with a thyroid disease, finds himself usually silent at bimonthly business meetings. He feels vaguely unhappy but never takes the time to identify all of the feelings he has in regard to these meetings. He becomes increasingly aware that he ends meeting days drinking too much in bars near his office. He arrives home to an angry wife who withdraws from him and leaves him to eat a cold dinner in an empty kitchen. He regards her as unfeeling and inconsiderate. Only in a very vague way does he make the connection between the business meetings, drinking, and the subsequent tension between himself and his wife.

If Andrew could decipher his automatic thoughts, he might discover that he is trapped by a belief that if he isn't going to sound erudite and impressively organized when he speaks, then he shouldn't talk. He is convinced that he couldn't bear the embarrassment of sounding stupid. So, he sits silently. Identifying his irrational beliefs can break open the way to heightened self-awareness. Deciphering the "code" of automatic thoughts will divulge feelings, needs, and expectations. In this way, Andrew might now identify his *feelings:* fear of looking stupid, awkwardness at public speaking, embarrassment at his lack of organization. He can admit his *needs:* to look bright, to be accepted by others, to be admired, to be successful. He can explore his *expectations:* "I'll be rejected if I don't sound prepared"; "If I do not appear bright, I will fail to get ahead"; "I'll make a fool of myself if I open my mouth"; "No one will understand how I feel about public speaking."

Exploration of his feelings, needs, and expectations will help Andrew to become aware of the destructive patterns of his behavior. Silence at meetings and excessive drinking are two behaviors that might well fulfill his fears of being rejected by both his employer and his wife.

Scripture maintains that "the truth will set you free."[1] The corollary is that erroneous thinking will keep us enslaved, not free to play, love, laugh, or genuinely succeed in being ourselves. Two of our greatest needs are to meet others in a satisfying and trusting way and to experience inner confidence and sense of worth. Two experts in cognitive psychology, Aaron Beck and Albert Ellis, delineate some of the false thinking that undermines our efforts to meet these profound human needs.

Beck describes the common false thoughts that sabotage meeting social needs:

1. "Any strange situation should be regarded as dangerous."
2. "A situation or a person is unsafe until proven to be safe."
3. "Strangers despise weakness."
4. "People will attack at a sign of weakness."

5. "If I am attacked, it will show that I appeared weak and socially inept."[2]

Programmed with such thoughts, we will find it impossible to engage in healthy, satisfying social interaction.

Virginia is plagued with chronic fatigue. She complains,

> I'm dragging myself from day to day, but I have to act like I'm not tired at work. I work for this design company where enthusiasm and energy are musts. It's kind of like we all represent our product. That's our company slogan. I'm afraid that I can't keep the act up anymore because I'm so exhausted. But I'm even more afraid that if I let them know what I'm going through it will mean the end of my job. I just wouldn't be accepted there in this lethargic state.

Virginia has decided that her employers are the enemy. They are ready to pounce and to reject. Her irrational thinking allows no trust in people whom she has enjoyed working with for nine years. They are deprived of an opportunity to express care, and Virginia is deprived of experiencing their compassion.

Albert Ellis focuses on irrational ideas that are commonly held and that threaten one's self-worth and independence. Typical ones are:

1. The idea that it is a dire necessity for an adult human being to be loved or approved of by virtually every significant other person in his community.
2. The idea that one should be thoroughly competent, adequate, and achieving in all possible respects if one is to consider oneself worthwhile.
3. The idea that it is easier to avoid than to face certain life difficulties and self-responsibilities."[3]

Idea No. 1 crushes initiative and independent behavior while enforcing stifling conformity. "What would the neighbors think?" replaces "What behavior would be satisfying and right for me?" as the criterion for behavior. Fear of "What will my parents think?" keeps a person from responsible personal reflection and authentic behavior. It is imperative to know one's needs and feelings, one's values and beliefs. Each authentic decision a person makes requires that he reflect on his needs and values and decide in a manner congruent with them, in a manner that is true to self. Concern with what others might think distracts a person from such reflection and such responsible behavior.

Denise, who has MS, faces a constant dilemma. On the one hand, she desperately wants sympathy for enduring the effects of MS. On the other, she dreads the thought of anyone knowing that she has MS.

> My husband's supervisor invited us to a concert next week. Instead of being thrilled at going to the symphony, I dread it. I feel so resentful that I'm in this position. I can't walk without losing my balance. My daughter said it looks like I'm drunk. When I lean on my husband's arm, I stay pretty steady. But what if he isn't nearby? What will I do? I don't want anyone to know that I have MS. I certainly don't want anyone to think I've been drinking. I think it's best that we skip events like this.
>
> I know my husband thinks I should just tell people that I have MS. I just don't think you should tell people something like this. You don't know what they'll do with it or who else they would tell. It's better to keep it to ourselves.

Denise's thinking makes what others might think more important than enjoyment of life. Her thinking, while leading to avoidance of social life and entertainment, also precludes expression of support and care. It also may inhibit her husband's life. The price she pays for her thinking is suffocatingly high.

Larry's faulty thinking leads to lack of self-worth. Larry, who has CMT, first came to therapy saying he was depressed.

He complained that his family considered him lazy and accused him of whining. At first glance Larry's family's judgments appeared accurate. He sat in the chair, his head down and his shoulders slumped. He admitted that he hadn't worked in six months and that he had given up on his job search. He spoke in a despondent tone.

> I feel miserable and I'm tired. My hands are always cold and my feet simply don't do what they're supposed to do. People expect me to continue to go on as if nothing is wrong. But everything is wrong. I don't walk as I used to and there is no way I can get a job in construction anymore. There's no way I'm going to get a job on a site. My family thinks I'm lazy. I'm not. I just don't have anything to offer anymore. I never went to college—or I ought to say I never finished. The only thing I'm good at is building, and that door is shut to me now.

Larry concludes that he has nothing to offer. His worth is totally dependent on working in construction. His irrational thinking defeats him.

Self-fulfilling Prophecies

Automatic irrational thoughts lead to self-defeating behavior. If a person believes that it is necessary for him to be loved or approved of by everyone, then he will strive to achieve this approval. The strategies he employs to reach this goal invariably lower his self-esteem and self-confidence, promote mistrust, and often lead to rejection by others.

Richard, a nineteen-year-old college sophomore, evidences such thinking and behavior. If someone needs help, Richard is always there. He is far happier giving than receiving. After a short time in therapy, Richard discovered that though he did genuinely enjoy taking care of others, he tended to do so at the expense of his own health. Crohn's disease had plagued him since he was fairly young, but few people outside of his immediate family knew of his illness. Richard's failure to disclose his Crohn's disease stemmed from feelings of embarrassment and shame. And these feelings in turn triggered his need to serve others rather than let others take care of him in any way. He had developed a pattern of relating that was based on pleasing others. His assertion that "I like to make people happy" failed to acknowledge a deeper reality, which would more truly be stated, "I like people to be happy because if they're pleased they'll like me."

Richard inevitably is taken advantage of in his relationships. He does too many favors, gives too many gifts, pursues others too vigorously. His lack of self-respect and self-worth makes it difficult for him to say no to others. These behaviors he rationalizes—"I like to be generous"— but the rationalization masks the truth of his feelings of inferiority. So Richard repeats self-denigrating behaviors and endures repeated rejections. Until he learns to admit his feelings and needs and to change his thinking and his behavior, Richard will be on a path to despair.

As Richard has been trapped by the lie that he needed to be loved by everyone, Maria, who suffers from Charcot-Marie-Tooth disease, was imprisoned by the belief that every new situation has to be dangerous. Maria is a slightly overweight forty-year-old woman who has never married and seldom dated. Maria's language in her first therapy session revealed her sad tendency to deceive herself regarding her true needs and feelings.

> I'm not the kind of person who just jumps into something, sight unseen. I like to check things out first. Maybe that's a fault, but I'm sorry, that's the kind of person I am.

Maria credited herself with a nature that is sensibly cautious and prudent. But beneath the self-justifying language, Maria was terribly lonely and unsure of herself. Her denied fears of the unfamiliar kept her from initiating new experiences, starting new relationships. She still lived at home with her parents, had kept the same cashier job for fifteen years, and kept her very limited social life to a few girl friends whom she had known for years. Her restricted life kept her from exploring new activities. Her irrational thinking and fearful behavior resulted in a lifestyle that confirmed her belief that newness was to be feared.

Every human being engages in irrational thinking. When we care deeply for someone our needs with regard to that person are heightened. We become vulnerable and in our vulnerability our thinking may become distorted. Or when we are unusually fearful we may surrender to irrational thoughts and imaginings. Chronic illness can certainly render the sufferer prone to such thinking. In the following chapter we look at different kinds of self-defeating irrational thinking, how this thinking is stirred by ICI, and what steps need to be taken to think in a rational, healthy manner.

11

Irrational Thinking and ICI

And in my hour of darkness
she'll be standing right in front of me,
speaking words of wisdom,
let it be.

The Beatles

We tend not to perform at our optimum level when we are not feeling well. The truth of that statement is self-evident when applied to mountain climbing. It might not be so evident when applied to thinking. Sickness makes us vulnerable. When we perceive ourselves to be weak, not in control, and threatened, our vulnerability can distort our thinking. In turn, distorted thinking can increase our sense of vulnerability.

Sandra is a successful real estate agent. Her income has been over $100,000 five years in succession. She is known by her colleagues as very bright, imaginative, "on the ball." Sandra was diagnosed with lupus five years previously. Her self-description during an exacerbation belies those qualities:

> I come from a fairly big family. I have two sisters and two brothers. They have all been mildly successful in their careers but I'm the only one who has really succeeded—though I've never believed that I could maintain the success. I am always uptight. A couple of years ago, I found I had lupus. Before that I had begun to feel more relaxed; I was even beginning to believe that I could

achieve without worrying. But with lupus, I am so often tired. Most of the time I don't have energy to get my work done very effectively. Lupus has made me more "uptight" than I ever was.

Last week I showed a house to a couple. They were very excited about the house and said they were so grateful that I had understood exactly what they needed. I was embarrassed that they were so grateful. After all, isn't a real estate agent supposed to tune in to what the client needs? The next day they called with a bid for the house; however, I had had a very bad night so when they called I was pretty distracted and I didn't take the figure in accurately. This is a very bad habit I have. A very bad habit. When I'm tired, I tend to let things slide rather than concentrate more. I don't develop habits like writing things down instead of committing them to memory.

In this case my bad habit could cause disastrous results. I called this couple's bid in at a figure of about $5,000.00 lower than they said. Can you believe I could make a mistake like that? I'm afraid to go into the office or to call these people. They'll be furious with me. I'm sure I'll lose the sale and these people will lose the house.

I have been debating for some time whether I should give up being a real estate agent entirely. I just don't feel well most of the time and I'm so scared that I will make mistakes more frequently. It's a sad thought for me because I'm not sure what else I could do. I have so-called people skills—but so what. You don't get a degree for being able to talk easily with people. You have to be able to produce, to make money.

Sandra manifests faulty thought processes that are characteristic of the vulnerable person's thinking. She underestimates her strengths, functioning on what psychiatrist Aaron T. Beck calls *minimization*. He refers to this kind of thinking as cognitive distortion.[1] Evidence of this self-deprecating thinking can be seen in her words:

>"I've never believed that I could maintain success."
>
>"I'm always uptight."
>
>"I was embarrassed that they were so grateful. After all, isn't a real estate agent supposed to tune in to what the client needs?"

She demeans herself and downplays her natural gifts for understanding her clients' needs. As much as she ignores her strengths, Sandra focuses on her weaknesses—a thought process that Beck identifies as *selective abstraction,* another cognitive distortion. She manifests this tendency to focus on her limits in her comment: "This is a very bad habit I have. A very bad habit. When I'm tired, I tend to let things slide rather than concentrate more. I don't develop habits like writing things down instead of committing them to memory." Sandra sums up her focus on her weaknesses by remarking, "I'm so scared that I will make mistakes more frequently."

Two other self-defeating cognitive distortions that Beck associates with the vulnerable person are *magnification,* exaggerating each mistake, and *catastrophizing,* concluding total disaster. Sandra's account demonstrates both behaviors. She magnifies her errors:

>"Can you believe I could make a mistake like that?"
>
>"I'm afraid to go into the office or to call these people."
>
>"In this case my bad habit could cause disastrous results."

She concludes total catastrophe:

>"They'll be furious with me."
>
>"I'm sure I'll lose the sale and these people will lose the house."
>
>"I have been debating for some time whether I should give up being a real estate agent entirely."
>
>"It's a sad thought for me because I'm not sure what else I could do."

Sandra is not thinking clearly. She is vulnerable in her sickness, and her thinking makes her more so. She is not thinking in a self-respecting, rational manner. Hers is the distorted thinking of someone who feels weak and worthless and who, by the way that she thinks, makes herself feel hopeless. Such thinking is common to persons with invisible chronic illness. How to confront and to change such thinking will be treated later in this chapter.

Faulty Assumptions

People suffering from ICI often hold as truths what are in actuality dangerous assumptions. These assumptions are often false and as such victimize the ICI patient. Fears of being unloved, unsuccessful, and out of control give rise to these faulty assumptions. The assumptions provoke irrational thinking in specific situations.

Faulty Love Assumptions
1. If I'm not healthy, I'm not really lovable.
2. I'm nothing unless I'm loved.
3. I'm not attractive if I'm sick.
4. I'm of no value if I can't do things for you.

Examples of Irrational Thinking
A. A woman has a partial hysterectomy to remove a diseased ovary caused by endometriosis. The surgery fails to relieve symptoms of severe pain. "How can my husband love me in this condition?"
B. A man becomes increasingly impotent from MS and is infrequently able to have intercourse.
   "No woman wants a man who can't make love."
C. A woman with lupus finds being in the sun dangerous. She refuses to participate in any outdoor activity.
   "People can't possibly want to be with me if I can only do things indoors. I feel like a scourge in my family."
D. A woman suffering from irritable bowel syndrome is invited to a summer cookout.

"I can't go and wear something summery. I feel totally ugly."

Faulty Success or Competence Assumptions

1. I'm worthless if I'm not successful. I can't be successful and sick.
2. I can't be a good mother if I can't always be available for my children.
3. I'm no use as a father if I can't provide for my family.
4. You can't be a good parent if you've harmed your child.

Examples of Irrational Thinking

A. A woman with chronic fatigue immune dysfunction syndrome has reluctantly rearranged her schedule and changed jobs to live with her chronic fatigue. "I feel worthless. They call this job low-stress—AKA dead-end."

B. A woman with multiple sclerosis finds herself depressed and contemplating divorce. Chronic fatigue keeps her from being her husband's companion in sports and other activities.

"How can I be a wife if I can't do anything he wants to do?"

C. A man who has Charcot-Marie-Tooth disease recently learned that his daughter probably has the disease. He rages at his wife, "I knew I should never be a father."

Faulty Control Assumptions

1. I can't tolerate not being in control.
2. I have to be perfect to be in control.
3. I can't bear this pain. I couldn't live the rest of my life with this pain.
4. I'd die if I were incontinent—I just couldn't handle the humiliation.

Examples of Irrational Thinking

A. A man who has been told that he probably has MS will not talk about the disease to his family.

"If I told my sister how scared I am, I would fall apart."

B. A woman with Crohn's disease breaks down and sobs uncontrollably when she realizes that she has made an error in a computer program.

"I have no room for mistakes; I'll be fired."

C. A woman with endometriosis who has grown up being told by her mother that men do not want to discuss menstruation and pain keeps her home so clean as to be sterile and is flawlessly organized.

"The only way I can live with myself is to be neat."

Feelings and Faulty Thinking

We have seen that being sick and vulnerable can affect the way that we think. Feelings themselves affect our thinking. Feeling very depressed certainly affects the way that we think about everything—an upcoming birthday, Christmas, the world situation. Feeling guilty affects our thoughts regarding our parents or children. Feeling sad colors our thoughts about events, as does feeling happy. One morning we might think that we can accomplish anything; another morning we might want to avoid the day itself. Feeling energetic, we think positively; feeling lonely and sad triggers very different thoughts.

It is important that we know our feelings and their effect on the way we think. It is especially important to realize that certain feelings can lead us to faulty thinking. Jack, for example, tends to feel guilt, and this guilt overwhelms his thinking.

I think the worst part of being sick is the guilt I feel. I was married three months when I had the first symptoms of MS. They were pretty mild. We went on a delayed honeymoon to Bermuda and it was a particularly hot summer. My speech was slurry and my right leg started to drag. It scared the hell out of my wife. Since that time I haven't had any major problems but I have had a lot of vague odd symptoms, which has created this subtle gloom over our lives all the time. I think I have really let my wife down. She had everything to look forward to and then this came in and took that away from her. Life seems grim.

Jack's guilt at having MS distorts his thinking. He has not only assumed responsibility for his wife's happiness but has also concluded that she is without joy and without hope due to his illness. Unless he realizes that he is assuming far more than might be valid, he will begin to act out his feelings by withdrawing. Such behavior could isolate him from his wife and indeed trigger in her the feelings that he has already ascribed to her.

Esther is prone to anxiety, a feeling that can easily distort her thinking. At this time Esther is suffering from an exacerbation of MS, which has affected her bowel control.

"What if . . ." is the way Esther frequently begins a sentence. She rarely reflects on her condition without contemplating a future event fraught with mishaps and failure. "What if I do decide to go out and I have an accident? What if no one I trust is there to help me? I'll be mortified. People will scorn me for not being more careful. It will be so humiliating." Her anxious, distorted thinking promotes increased anxiety.

Emotions need to be brought into awareness and their impact on thinking needs to be acknowledged. Particularly for the ICI patient, feelings can fluctuate rapidly and intensely. With awareness, these feelings need not distort thought processes. Without awareness, they will do just that, thereby fanning the feelings that gave rise to the thought and leading to destructive behaviors.

Confronting Feelings and Irrational Thoughts

When you contemplate situations in your life that provoke feelings of fear, guilt, anxiety, sadness, anger, and shame, try to *state the thoughts* that go through your mind in these situations. Now ask yourself, "What is the evidence to support such thinking?" For example, the man growing impotent with MS is asked for evidence to support his thought, "No woman wants a man who can't make love." The woman with lupus who must avoid the sun is asked for evidence to support her conclusion that "People can't possibly want to be with me if I can only do things indoors." Usually no present evidence can be given and the client is led to see the irrational, self-defeating nature of the thought. Even if some evidence is proffered, other explanations are explored. For example, the woman who is convinced that her husband does not want her because she can no longer play sports with him can learn to realize that his irritation on golf days is due not to her failure to join him but to the self-pitying and angry tone she displays at those times.

Source of Irrational Thinking

Challenge your irrational thinking not only by asking yourself to justify your thinking but also by asking where these thoughts come from. It is intellectually satisfying and eventually liberating to identify the source of thinking. This exploration leads into the past, into childhood, into present relationships. Assumptions that seemed like absolute truths can be unmasked and seen as stemming from mother or father—and for them the "truth" was often not reflective of happiness or success. The assumption that one must be "totally competent to be worthwhile" might have governed a person's father, but it probably didn't make him competent and it surely didn't foster in him feelings of self-worth. The notion that we are lovable to the degree that we are successful is a sad and untrue message propagated in sad, humorless families. Yet it is in our families and in early, repetitive experiences that we develop the subconscious mental structures with which we define ourselves and our basic attitudes.

These basic mind sets toward the world are ones of trust or distrust, hostility or friendliness, enthusiasm or depression. From these subconscious schema come automatic thoughts. Given a poor table in a restaurant, one person (hostile schema) will think, "They did this on purpose," and argue. Another (depressive) schema will think, "This always happens to me," and feel hopelessly resigned. Buying a house, a person with an anxious schema will think of all the problems that might make this choice unwise, while a person with an enthusiastic schema will picture all of the joy and satisfaction this house will provide. These schema were developed without conscious reflection in our childhood. They need to be consciously explored and examined since they are a powerful source of automatic thoughts. Insight into the source of our irrational thinking does not guarantee freedom from its grip, but it is a step toward loosening it.

Forming Healthy and Rational Thinking

"The truth will set you free." Lies tie us up in knots. The irrational thoughts that govern us are really lies, lies that we tell ourselves over and over in situation after situation. "I will never be happy," "No one could really love me," "I know I'll be fired"—all are lies. These untrue statements keep us anxious, depressed, hopeless. They predict our attitude and behavior; also, as we have seen, they are self-fulfilling. Beneath these statements lies their history—we have to dig down to discover their genesis and then challenge their validity.

Andy, who struggles with irritable bowel syndrome, is a very successful publishing executive. His income has been in six figures for over ten years. Yet the lie that keeps driving him to overwork at the expense of family life and leisure is, "Work now and salt it away. It can all be taken away in an instant." It was rather easy for Andy to trace the origins of the warning. His parents were children of the Depression and Andy grew up on a small farm in Wisconsin. Over and over as a boy he saw his parents deny themselves any luxury. Money had to be saved. A drought could wipe them out. Being frugal was the only way to stave off disaster.

"Better safe than sorry." Even though Andy has hundreds of thousands of dollars saved and has provided his wife and three girls with an expensive home, he rules the house, rules the budget, limits expenses, and avoids vacations, as though penury could be the cost of any "extravagance."

Andy's thinking has little to do with present reality. Once the origins of the thought have been established and the consequences of such thinking have been identified (loss of family life, frustration of wife and children at lack of family vacations and pleasures, cost to his body and psyche), the challenge then is to think and to act more in conformity with the financial facts and more in accord with his and his family's needs.

It is a good idea to keep a notebook that is divided into columns. The first column is for the incident or situation that provokes the thought. In the second column, the client records the irrational thought; in the third, the emotional effect of this thought; and in the fourth, the behavior that is triggered. For example, Andy's predicament is outlined below:

Situation	Irrational Thought	Resulting Feeling	Resulting Behavior
Possible family vacation.	We cannot afford it. The money it would cost could be saved and will some-day keep hunger from the door.	Hurt at the family's lack of appreciation and understanding. Resentment and loneliness. Discouragement.	Angry family arguments. Daughters distant and withdrawn.

You can see that by recording the events and reactions, you can gain greater awareness of irrational thoughts and their destructive power. Then challenge yourself to express the *truth*. This truth starts with a feeling and is followed by the reason for the feeling.

Feeling	*Reason*
I feel anxious at the prospect of spending money for a family vacation.	I fear that the vacation will be expensive and will damage our financial security.

Once the truth of the feeling and the reason for the feeling are admitted, you can explore the truth further to see if the feeling and the reason are reasonable. You must ask yourself, "Do the feeling and reason match the present reality?" In this case, Andy is nondefensive enough to see that his thoughts and feelings are conditioned from childhood and are not reasonable guides to rational behavior in the present.

Carolyn, a freshman in college, provides the material for the next example. Carolyn had suffered from chronic fatigue for a year. Despite her condition, she planned to continue in school. After several discussions with her doctor, Carolyn developed a plan to make attending classes feasible. The plan included periodic rests during the school day. One month into the semester she reported her progress to her doctor. He found her predictably tired, but far more exhausted and discouraged than he expected. Carolyn admitted that she had not taken rests during the day. "It's too embarrassing to tell people that I have to lie down. They will think that I'm a dork—like pathetic." When prompted to explore her thinking in the way we described previously, Carolyn explained the following:

Situation	*Thought*	*Resulting Feeling*	*Resulting Behavior*
Needing a resting place on campus.	People will not like me and respect me if I am different.	Embarrassed, inadequate, vulnerable.	Failing to do what is best for her body, which increased her fatigue and triggered discouragement.

When encouraged to look further into her thoughts and feelings, Carolyn discovered the following:

Feeling	*Reason*
I am embarrassed to ask for a place to lie down.	I am afraid of not being liked or respected.

When Carolyn states her feelings and needs out loud, she realizes that embarrassment is proving costly to her health. She also concludes that, though she naturally wants to be liked and respected, the kind of people whom she would want as friends would not be so crass and insensitive as to condemn her for needing rest.

The following example concerns Joan, an ICI patient whose husband's company is planning a summer outing.

Situation	*Irrational Thought*	*Resulting Feeling*	*Resulting Behavior*
Husband's company outing.	I can't go because I couldn't join in the activities and I would feel like a fool.	Depression, sadness, resentment.	Staying home, feeling sorry for self. Argument with husband.

With reflection, Joan is able to give a more accurate description of her feelings and the reason behind them.

Feeling	*Reason*
I feel afraid to go to the outing.	I am afraid that everyone would be playing volleyball or tennis and I would be all by myself feeling lonely and awkward.

By stating her feelings and thoughts so clearly, Joan might realize that not everyone will be playing these games. She might see that she can be a cheering spectator without being a pariah. She might conclude that her need in this situation is that her husband be emotionally and often physically connected to her during the event. When her true feelings and needs have been admitted to herself and possibly shared with her husband, then she will be freed from the lock of the previous irrational thinking and feel and act differently.

The way you think governs the way you feel and guides the way you live. You talk to yourself all day and often all night long. If you are telling yourself untrue thoughts, then you are poisoning the way you feel about yourself, about your illness, about others, about your life. Your life will reflect the toxic untruths you feed yourself. Become aware of what you are saying to yourself. Challenge the veracity of what you are saying. "This above all, to thine own self be true."[2] Perhaps you say in prayer, "Give us this day our daily bread" and then in the next breath bite into unnourishing lies about yourself. A priest friend of ours put it this way,

> If the call to renewal means anything, it means that God is asking us to draw more deeply from those resources which generate in us enthusiasm, joy, a feeling of worth— all qualities of abundant life. We are called to eat the "living bread" rather than feed on those debilitating experiences which engender discouragement, loss of energy, a sense of futility—all marks of slow death.

12

Using Imagery to Confront Irrational Thinking

For oft when on my couch
I lie in vacant or in pensive mood
They flash upon that inward eye
That is the bliss of solitude
And then my heart with gladness fills
And dances with the daffodils.

Wordsworth

A picture is worth a thousand words and is probably a thousand times more powerful. Paul first became aware of the power of imagery on a beautiful July morning in suburban St. Louis. He had stopped at his sister's in-laws' home to swim and have breakfast before driving on to the clinic where he worked. He described the experience.

I was thoroughly enjoying the clear blue water, the fresh morning air and warm sun. Yet, I was frustrated, because I was trying to execute a jack-knife from the diving board. Each time I dove, I would bend my body and then straighten to enter the water. Over and over I did the same dive. It felt okay, but I was not bending all the way to touch my toes—not doing a jack-knife. I'd tell myself, "Now, this time, bend totally, do it," but then I would repeat the same incomplete dive as the previous one. Just then my sister's mother-in-law, Betty, called from the house that breakfast was ready. They were moving to Boston the next day. It was my last chance to do one final dive. I remember stopping myself on the board and picturing exactly what a perfect jack-knife would look like. I pictured the body bending totally, the head tucked between the arms, which were fully extended to touch the pointed toes. I hit the board firmly with my feet, sprang up high from the board and did the perfect jack-knife I had been attempting. It was such a strongly felt experience of the power of an image.

We can't do what we can't picture. And we can't be what we can't imagine. That's the reason we need role models, people whom we can view in the way they perform simple actions or live their lives. Swiss ski instructors have always known the power of the image. They do not give long verbal instructions about how to stand, how to turn, where to hold the hands, or how to weight and unweight the skis. They simply say, "Follow me." The skier learns by watching. The image of the expert instructor is constantly committed to the mind of the student. The image teaches more powerfully than verbal instruction.

A golf pro we know uses videotape to teach her pupils by way of images. She tapes the student and allows him to look at himself swinging the club. Then, on a split screen, she projects a professional golfer, like Ian Woosnam or Fred Couples, swinging. The aspiring golfer sees himself, sees the professional, and sees the difference. Other sports and various skills are now taught by way of seeing and imagining. Books like *Inner Tennis* and *Inner Skiing* teach by focusing on the function of the imagination in acquiring skills. Good skiers picture the slalom course in their minds and imagine how they will start, how they will flash low past the gates, and how they will finish. Golf and tennis stars picture their shots. The imagination leads the way to desired performance.

In Chapter 10 we demonstrated how irrational thinking undermines performance. "I can't do it" is the shortest, surest prescription for failure. Much irrational thinking is connected unwittingly to negative images. While you are saying, "I'm not attractive; he'd never notice me," you are undoubtedly picturing an unflattering you and a terribly flattering him, a him who in all his handsome grandeur sweeps past you, all eyes on him while his eyes are certainly not on you. When you are thinking, "I can't possibly accept the position—not with my health," you are probably having images of yourself exhausted during a meeting or unable to control shaking hands when delivering a report. Your pessimistic images connect with your irrational thinking to defeat you. Instead, you can learn to use your images to defeat such thinking.

Tammie suffers from fibromyalgia and from depressive negative thinking. When she came to see us, this twenty-eight-year-old waitress talked and felt as though her life was over. During a session when she was complaining of all the things she could no longer do, we stopped her and encouraged her to describe the images she was having as she talked. Her response painted a somber picture.

"I see myself in my apartment in my bedroom."

"Are the lights out?" we asked.

"Yeah, I guess so. Or it is very gloomy. I'm by myself. My friends are out canoeing, laughing, splashing around."

"What else do you picture?"

"I picture them playing softball. Running, hitting the ball. They're having a great time."

"Where are you?"

"I'm at home, not doing anything."

"Other images?"

"They're having a picnic. They're eating chicken, drinking beer."

"And what picture do you have of yourself?"

"Still in bed, probably trying to go to sleep."

It wasn't difficult for Tammie to see how her images made her so miserable. We asked her to create images of herself doing things she enjoyed.

"I'm sitting with some friends listening to old '60s records."

"What else?"

"We're talking, laughing, drinking some wine."

"Create some other images of you doing things you enjoy."

"I'm reading a good book in a comfortable chair and having something to eat. I'm knitting some baby clothes for my sister's baby. I'm listening to some Spanish tapes and repeating back the lesson."

Tammie has started to use her imagination to picture what she could do to enjoy herself rather than allow negative images of what she couldn't do to dominate her moods. People with ICI have to be careful to fight off images that portray them as being unable to do what they formerly enjoyed. Instead, they need to focus on images of what they can do. Henrietta Aladjem, author of *In Search of the Sun,* told us in an interview that when her mind is tired, she cleans her closet. Another day, when she is feeling creative, she writes. She bends with reality like a tree bending with the wind. The person with ICI needs to use her imagination to lead her realistically to satisfying activity. She must combat those images that portray her as helpless, hopeless, crippled, and alone.

Making Movies

As Hollywood has demonstrated, moving pictures have a power and influence all their own. Our minds are constantly producing short movies—fantasies that avoid reality, or happy-ending ones that encourage us to initiate and to take roles, or false films that intensify our irrational thinking. In the example described in the last chapter of the woman afraid to attend her husband's company outing, the client fanned her irrational thinking by producing, directing, and starring in a sad melodrama. In the mind's film, the client is sitting alone while others play. She has awkwardly declined invitations to join in and now experiences humiliating loneliness. Sounds of people playing tennis, having fun, and laughing taunt her. She wishes to disappear but is trapped. The film is as fraudulent as her thinking.

Image and thought, joined together by fear, threaten her well-being.

Become more aware of the images and "movies" that you create. Again, the path to these images begins with *feelings*. For people with ICI the feelings are often sadness, fear, helplessness, powerlessness, and anger. Once the feelings and images are clear, you can edit the film more in accord with reality. If, prompted by anxiety, you picture yourself being fired for making a mistake, we encourage you to change the scene to one that shows your boss correcting you for the error while you respond sensibly. If you are imagining that your husband is disgusted with you for having an exacerbation, we challenge you to create a film more in conformity with his confusion and love. Instead of picturing him rejecting you, you can form images of him expressing his frustration that you are in a weakened condition. Imagine yourself listening to him with understanding. Imagine him softening and the two of you embracing.

The following "movie-making" exercises are designed to assist you to become more proficient in creating the kinds of movie images that alleviate anxiety and a sense of helplessness and promote greater confidence and sense of control.

Situation #1: THE DOCTOR'S APPOINTMENT

Take One

You have a doctor's appointment and are afraid that he will be suspicious and lack understanding.

1. Describe the movie scene that you are creating. Exaggerate it into a worst-case scenario.
2. What does the office look like through the eyes of fear? Be specific and create the scene.
3. How do you look? Again, be specific with details.
4. How do you feel? If your inner voice were being heard in a voice-over, what would you be saying?

5. What does the doctor look like? What is his expression?
6. What does the doctor say? Remember to exaggerate.
7. What do you do? Again, exaggerate.

Take Two

Shoot the scene over. This time, be different in the starring role. Look right at the doctor. Let him stay distant and suspicious, but you be different. Confront him about his anger or criticism. Listen to him, but be strong and confident. Exaggerate your story a bit.

1. Does the office look the same as in the first scene? If it is different, how?
2. Do you look different? How? Be specific.
3. How do you feel?
4. How does the doctor look and what does he say?
5. What do you say and do? Be strong. Be in command of yourself and of the situation. Be specific.

Take Three

Redo the scene, making it closer to reality. At the same time, be the way you would like to be.

1. What does the office look like? Be confident as you view the scene. Be perceptive and even critical.
2. How do you look? How are you dressed? Look the way you want to look, the way you want to be seen.
3. How do you feel? Be confident. You are hiring the doctor. He needs your help to be effective.
4. How does the doctor look? What is his facial expression?
5. What does the doctor say?
6. What do you say? Remember to play the part with natural, graceful confidence, maybe even friendly wit. Say what you really want to say.
7. How does the scene end? Give the scene a realistic but happy ending.

The purpose of the exercise is to increase your awareness of how anxiety can trigger images that frighten you and sap your confidence. The exercise can help you to use your creative imagination to prepare yourself for anxiety-arousing situations by creating success in which you are more in control of yourself, more able to be the you that you wish to be.

Situation #2: VACATION WITH FRIENDS

Take One

You are planning to go on vacation with your family or with friends, but you are afraid that you might suffer an exacerbation. Shoot the movie as a worst-case scenario nightmare. Include cast of characters, setting, onset of illness, disastrous consequences of the decision to go.

Take Two

You do get sick on the trip but you handle yourself well. You admit your illness openly. You are heard and lovingly supported. Be specific with details regarding actions, facial expressions, words spoken. Be an active director.

Final Take

This time imagine the vacation without an exacerbation. Direct the scene filled with moments of enjoyment, relatively good health, and sensible care of yourself.

We waste great amounts of energy imagining the worst that can happen to us. We seldom go further in these imaginings to see ourselves handling even the worst possibility with grace, confidence, and dignity. We stop the movie at the crisis point, with ourselves as losers. We encourage you to keep your imagination's camera running until you like the way you are acting, no matter how difficult the situation. Remember, you can't do what you can't picture.

Situation #3: HOLIDAY TIME

Take One

A major holiday is approaching and a lot has to be done in preparation. Direct a short, tragic movie that portrays your worst fears. Again, remember to provide as many details as you, as a creative director, can employ. Who are the characters? How are they dressed? What do they say? Where are the scenes set? What happens? What goes awry? How do you feel?

Take Two

Redo the scene. In this scene you are still overwhelmed, but you ask for and receive help. Be realistic.

Final Take

Finally, redirect the movie into a happy-ending celebration of a wonderful holiday. Picture the way you want to be. Be specific. Make it good.

If you suffer from chronic illness, you can panic at holiday times or at any time that demands energy and enthusiasm. Unconsciously, you can begin to entertain crushing images. But with imagination you can picture the event the way you would like it to happen. You don't have to be a martyr or a saint. You can delete from the script whatever would be too much for you. You can work quietly. You can ask for help. You can picture a peaceful time. Making that time happen is more in your power than you might think.

Idealized Self-Image

Illness can be very hard on self-image. As we have discussed earlier, it is not easy to have a positive image of yourself when you feel no energy and no sparkle and when your confidence has been eroded by self-doubt and pain. In his book, *In the Mind's Eye,*[1] Arnold Lazarus discusses the concept of an idealized self-image as a step toward greater self-esteem and describes several steps in this process:

- Relax. Then picture yourself the way you would like to be. See in yourself qualities and behaviors that are not at all impossible for you to achieve. Be specific. Picture yourself walking into a room, talking to a friend, all the while manifesting qualities of confidence, grace, and caring, being the self that you want to be. Be specific in imagining the way you walk, talk, listen, move.
- Ask yourself how you ordinarily see yourself that could keep you from being your ideal self. Then determine what you have to change in order to realize your ideal self.
- We tend to remember our mistakes and to play them over and over in our minds. We can be our best selves more confidently when we recall our achievements, our best moments, happy incidents. We should dwell on these times.
- We have to carry over these good feelings and apply them to whatever we are doing at the moment.
- Finally, recall your ideal self frequently, especially before threatening situations. Picture yourself the way you want to be, then enter the room, call the doctor, address the group. Be all that you can be, letting your images lead you.

Fay, a thirty-two-year-old stockbroker with lupus, used the idealized self-image approach to discard a poor self-image that was hampering her well-being, personally as well as professionally. Despite being slim, educated, and attractive, Fay viewed herself in a dismal light, and her behavior, especially at work, reflected this image. She wore no makeup, was never satisfied with her hair, and felt awkward around the men in her office. She was aware that either she talked too much or she was shyly silent. Often she accused herself of being rather silly and frequently made self-deprecating remarks, such as, "I'll never get it right," or "I'm sorry for taking your time."

Determined to change, Fay formulated an idealized self-image as an attractive woman whose appearance was enhanced by light makeup. In her mind's picture she wore tasteful, fashionable clothes. She formed an image of being poised, confident, reserved but friendly. She decided that she had to make changes in her hair style, her clothes, her makeup, the manner in which she spoke. She knew that she had to stop self-denigrating remarks and to talk less when she was nervous.

After resolutely determining to change, Fay looked and acted like the woman she had always had the potential of being. She was promoted and shortly afterward changed firms, receiving another boost in salary. "This job," she said, "I will start with the image I want to be. They haven't seen the me I was and they won't."

Images of Hope

Possibly the most powerful use of the imagination for the person tormented by exacerbations of ICI is its ability to speed back in time and forward into the future. In this way, the imagination can place the suffering in context. There was a yesterday without pain. You can remember it, picture it, enjoy it. You can imagine a tomorrow in which the pain will have subsided. You do not need to be crushed under the suffocating present. The mentally disturbed often suffer intense depression and despair because their imaginations have been distorted, so that they cannot imagine beyond their present state. They have no hopeful images to enable them to wait for better times and lighter feelings. The person sick with ICI must develop his imagination and learn to form images of hope.

When you are in pain, you tend to picture a future in which you are handicapped or in persistent agony. But that image is not a true picture of the future—it is simply an extension of the present. You must learn to picture yourself with pain remitted and see yourself peacefully playing with your children, enjoying your partner, walking quietly in the woods. These images are usually more congruent with your past and more truthful about your future. Everyone needs images of hope. But such images are difficult to form when you are feeling anxiety and pain. Practice in relatively serene times to relish happy memories. Like Wordsworth, the Romantic poet, let these images "flash upon this inward eye which is the bliss of solitude." Learn to form images of the future that show you content, caring for those you love, performing activities that you enjoy.

Regina, who suffers from premenstrual syndrome, describes her image-making this way.

> I have images of myself feeling the pain enter my body and I'm lying in bed curled into a ball. My family is looking at me critically and with disdain. Then I try to imagine myself heading toward those two weeks of predictable pain with serenity. My two little girls are playing on the floor by a big comfortable chair where I sit wrapped in a big woolly blanket. I have a cup of tea on a table nearby and I'm reading a great, entrancing novel.

With effort, practice, and mental discipline, you can learn to control your imagination and to bring your mental pictures more into the service of the truth and mental health. The goal of learning to think and imagine rationally and truthfully is to know and to appreciate ourselves and the people in our lives. It is to know the truth and be freed by the truth of our fears and self-dislike. It is to live more deeply in peace and to give peace to those around us by relating truthfully and lovingly. Such a goal is worth all of the effort and discipline required. It is a goal that makes life rich in possibility and hope.

13

Living Your Story

All the world's a stage,
And all the men and women merely players;
They have their exits and their entrances;
And one man in his time plays many parts.

Shakespeare

Our thoughts and our images come together in the narratives of stories that we live by. Each of us unconsciously chooses stories early in our lives that shape and give meaning to our existences. We are the central actors in our narrative, a story that tells us who we are and how we should live. It tells us what we believe and what we value, whether we will marry and what kind of work we will do. Mandie's story features her as a star:

> I always thought that I was special and different from my brothers and sister. One of my brothers was the athlete and my sister was the brain, but I was always special, like the star in the family. My father used to call me "Princess." I used to fantasize being a princess in court or a star actress greeting her public. I always had a big part if not the lead in school productions. Then, after college, I came to New York. My life was a whirl of acting classes, dance classes, modeling, and a couple of parts in plays. But then, boom, chronic fatigue hit. My world collapsed. I tried for months to push myself but after a while I just couldn't. It's like my life is over.

Mandie's life is not over but her story needs to be revised. Mandie's story of being a star has shaped her life, directed her decisions concerning everything, from place of residence, to the role men are allowed to play in her life, to the type of clothes she wears, to the kind of low-calorie food she can eat. The story has provided meaning, motivation, even identity. Now chronic fatigue threatens to wipe out this meaning, this identity, this story. Mandie still needs to stand out. This need is not bad. But the story's plot has to be changed to help her meet her needs and live in a satisfying way while coping with chronic fatigue. Through counseling, she is understanding herself more deeply and learning to accept the limits that her illness enforces. This process of adapting to ICI is very difficult and very slow. It demands great patience. For months Mandie refused to accept the fact that she needed to change. She dragged herself through dance classes and exhausted herself with exercise and auditions. It was agony to continue her activities, but that agony seemed more bearable than the prospect of never acting again.

Mandie's adjustment was made more difficult by her fear of disappointing others. She described this dimension:

> I couldn't stand the thought of letting down the people who had stood behind me for years. My father had boasted about me and brought a group from his club to see me when I had a part on Broadway. My mother drove me to a zillion classes before I could drive and sat there waiting hour after hour. My agent's a honey who deserved that I make it big. You don't just disappoint yourself, you let so many people down. That's been hell.

Mandie is gradually letting go of her dream of being a Broadway star. She doesn't talk any more about how long it will be before she can go back. Now she is trying to meet her needs in other ways. She has moved back to Memphis and is trying to believe and to accept her parents' love and support. She has begun to teach a small acting class. She is trying to learn that she is special even when she is not in the spotlight.

Alisa's story was shaped, as were all of our stories, by

early life experiences. Her mother died on Alisa's fourth birthday. Her father, an emotionally remote and cold man, remarried a strong, self-willed woman who had three children from a previous marriage. Alisa grew up feeling very alone, very unloved. Her story is Cinderella but the young man whom she married to escape her home was no prince. Very early in the marriage she realized that he was unfaithful and cruel. So she remained "unloved and alone."

Like Cinderella, Alisa coped with her unhappiness with hard work. She also spent hours in artistic activity, becoming very skillful in various crafts. But lupus began to close off her escape routes of solitary work and crafts. She had no relief from illness and no one to lean on for support.

Her story is a sad one. In it she is abandoned by her true love, her mother, ignored and mistreated by the key people in her life, father, stepmother, stepbrothers and sisters, and then by her husband. She learns not to trust in love and reinforces the learning with her poor choice of a husband. She lives basically alone, surrendering herself emotionally to no one. She expects only hurt from others. Only her pets, with whom she is safe, receive her tenderness and love. Her time and energy are spent in creative work, but the onset of lassitude from lupus threatened her activities, and in the dependency that her fatigue forced on her, she came face to face with her loneliness and self-hatred. In despair, she attempted suicide. Her attempted suicide brought her to therapy.

Now Alisa is painstakingly rewriting her story. Slowly she is learning to respect herself and to trust others. She has divorced her husband, grown increasingly closer to her children, has let herself love and be loved by them, and for the first time in her life has genuine friends. Such change has required several years of effort and demanded great courage. She has had to learn to communicate her deepest feelings, to listen to the feelings of others, and to trust the respect and love that others have for her. Bit by bit her creativity is becoming a rich source of self-expression, as well as providing an income. Her crafts and art work are exquisite and command good prices. In Alisa's new story she is no longer alone and unloved. There is still no prince, but maybe she doesn't need one.

Each of us lives out a story that has informed us about our identity, our values, and our meaning in life. The story is influenced by our families, our culture, our religion, and our ethnic origin. The story might conform to external reality and it might not. If in my story I am to be a famous singer and yet I can't hold a note, the discrepancy will defeat me. My story might cast me in the role of Florence Nightingale or of Jesus Christ; pursuing this role, I might accomplish great good or have a breakdown trying to be perfect. My story might be colored by the guilt or gloom of my family or ethnic background with the consequence that I am not free to be happy or to be peaceful but am condemned to play the role of martyr or victim. My story might have no tolerance for the weakness of illness. Our task is to identify our stories and to revise them if necessary so that they free us to love ourselves as we are, to accept others as they are, and to enjoy life in as wholesome a way as possible. There is some destiny in all of our stories, but we all have the freedom and responsibility to shape our stories as we live them.

Some stories have to be radically altered due to invisible chronic illness. For others the arrival of illness fits too readily into their stories. Gene's story features him as a victim. His father abandoned his mother, brothers, and himself when he was twelve. Gene's mother seems to have been drinking before her husband's departure. Afterward, she became increasingly dependent on alcohol. Gene's brothers were older and soon moved away. Gene learned to take care of himself. He did well in school and always worked, often at more than one job. His memories are unhappy ones. He remembers fearing his mother's mood swings and keeping distant from her. In recounting his story he mentioned frequently how hard he had worked and how alone he had been.

Gene received a scholarship to the Naval Academy, where, again, he succeeded academically. He had an outstanding naval career until it was curtailed by Crohn's disease. His marriage broke up two years after he was diagnosed with the disease. In his first therapy session, Gene summed up the marriage on the theme of unfairness, "I gave 90 percent, all I wanted was some giving on her part. It was so unfair. I was totally taken advantage of. She is not going to find someone who will give like I did. She had real nerve to walk out on me when I'm sick. I can't believe it.

Gene's illness fits his script. Gene has felt like a victim all his life—a victim of his mother's alcoholism, a victim of his brothers' departure, a victim of his father's abandonment, a victim of his wife's selfishness, and now a victim of Crohn's disease. If Gene is going to find and succeed in a relationship that he has already begun with a caring and attractive woman, he is going to have to overcome his readiness to experience himself as unfairly victimized. Using his intelligence and his willingness to work hard in therapy, Gene has identified his victim role and even learned to laugh at himself when we humorously tease him about his self-serving tales. Between therapy sessions he records in his journal instances where he catches himself indulging in blame of others for not giving him the recognition that he "deserves." Such self-serving thinking is automatic and has been part of his lifelong victim role. Changing the thinking, changing the image of himself, changing his story will be very challenging. But he is making steps and he is motivated.

All too often we live out our stories without reflection, without choice, as though we were handed a script when we come into the world on which our role, our lives, our actions are all printed. In the next chapter we will discuss how to identify our story and the role we play in it. First we will see how we take all of life's events and make them into stories to fit into our own overall story. Then we will talk about ICI as a life event that becomes part of our story.

Events as Stories

We have talked about our whole lives as narratives, that is, stories that we choose to live that shape as well as explain our lives. We make stories also of events in our lives, and we do so for the same reason that we make our lives stories—to give meaning and value to the event, as well as to fit the event into our life story. Joan, the mother of three, told us this story about the birth of her son, now four years old.

It's always seemed to me that Bobby chose us and came to us. We had decided not to have any more children after our first son and daughter. Both of us thought two children was just right. Then three years later Bobby came. He has always had the sweetest and most loving disposition. And he's so independent. I know that he chose us to bring his joy and light into our lives. It's hard to explain but I really feel it.

Joan's story of Bobby springs right from her. The story is as unplanned as Bobby's birth. It explains his unexpected arrival and it gives his birth meaning. Bobby wasn't planned—*he* did the choosing. Moreover, Joan does not see herself or her husband as the loving and sweet ground from which such a good-natured child could grow. He came, thus, independently to bring these qualities into the family. He was not chosen, but he was needed. The story also explains Bobby's independent personality—he even chose when and to whom he was to be born.

Kelly, an attractive twenty-eight-year-old client with endometriosis, came in for her weekly therapy session with the story of a car accident. Kelly has been taking control of her life, learning to separate herself from her family, where she plays the role of the independent but angry daughter. She is furious with her mother for her depressive, listless way of living and has been caught in a futile effort to change her. Weekly she returns home to visit and to engage in angry rebellious behavior with her mother and sullen exchanges with her father. The following is part of the story that she told.

It was so stupid. I had been at my brother's house for his baby's christening, for which my mother did nothing. As usual at family events, I drank too much. I'm stubborn so I was determined to drive myself home. The road was dark and as I came up over a hill, I must have hit a slick spot. I lost control for a second. The car jumped over the curb, side-swiped a tree, then spun back onto the road. I pulled over and stopped. I sat there shaking and then drove home very slowly. God was reaching down and shaking me. I'm changing and respecting myself. But he was saying, "Stop drinking, change the way you are with your family, let go and stop trying to hurt yourself." Believe me I'm listening. I'm not going to drink at all and I'm determined to change. It was an $800 lesson, but that's okay. It will be worth it.

Kelly's accident is for her a story of reckless behavior triggered by the anger and frustration she feels in her family. But it is also a story of redemption. God has "warned" her to take a major step in redirecting her life. His warning complements the insights she is acquiring in therapy and reinforces the determination she has been nurturing to change her life. For someone else the same incident could become a story of being a failure, or a story of being lucky, or a story that confirms a conviction that life is futile. For Kelly it is a sobering story, but one that gives hope. She is not alone. God cares for her and is encouraging her to live more rationally and more caring of herself. The accident for Kelly becomes a love story—God's love for her and her need to love herself.

What story we create regarding an event shapes the event, gives it meaning, and gives us attitudes, feelings, and ways of coping with it. Invisible chronic illness is a major event in the lives of those it affects. It can become a story of the futility of trying to be happy or of courage in the presence of adversity. How it is storied is our next focus.

Invisible Chronic Illness as
a Narrative

Roberta first sensed that something was wrong with her when she discovered a strange rash on her face. Then other symptoms appeared. She lost a lot of hair and felt unusual aches and pains. A blood test revealed that she had lupus. Roberta was devastated. The diagnosis felt to her like a public condemnation. She felt humiliation and shame. She felt branded by the word "lupus" and began immediately to try to expunge the word from herself. She made repeated visits to her physician and insisted that he schedule new blood tests and check for other illnesses. She told no one but her husband of the diagnosis, adamant that no one, not even the grown children, needed to know. If she feared that she might feel sick, she would avoid any social invitations. If she feared that the rash would reappear on her face, she would stay at home for weeks. Roberta's illness was not to be acknowledged or witnessed. For her, it was a shameful stigma that, if ignored, might seem not to exist.

Roberta has translated her illness into a sad story of shamefaced denial. Her illness is a humiliating indictment that she is not perfect—an indictment so threatening to her identity that it must be denied. What did Roberta need to do to rewrite this story? She had to learn to accept her lupus as an illness, not as a source of shame. She had to recognize other areas of her life that she had hidden or denied—the failure of her only child, her son, to get into Yale and her husband's failure to become senior law partner in his firm. She had to explore her background to discover the sources of her story. For Roberta, this meant tracing back to her mother's alcoholism, the origin of her emphasis on the importance of keeping all family matters private and of keeping up appearances at all costs. She had to learn the meaning of self-acceptance—to believe genuinely that she is sensitive, caring, funny, and insightful. She had to acknowledge the unreasonable expectation that she had placed on herself—the demand to be perfect. She had to learn how to share her feelings with others—openly and with trust. These steps to creating a new, more authentic story were painstakingly taken one at a time.

Invisible chronic illness, like all other events in our lives, is made into a story; that is, it is given a meaning and value, given even a kind of life of its own. ICI can be punishment for our sins and excesses, an enemy to be conquered, another proof that life is hopeless, an excuse for nonachievement. It can be an intimate, difficult, never faraway companion with whom we can learn to live. It can be a cross given by God that, if carried courageously, can transform our lives. It can be a painful life experience that forces us to grow as we learn to cope and endure.

Mark first met multiple sclerosis with rage. It threatened his love of sports, even his optimistic, happy way of life. Mark was twenty-eight when MS interrupted his life as a marathon runner. He had run in all of the major marathons and was moving into the ranks of world-class long-distance runners when MS forced him to stop running. After initial periods of anger and depression, Mark became active in the MS associations and activities. MS provided Mark with a new mission—a route to inspire hope for those suffering multiple sclerosis and to promote understanding of the illness.

Despite his illness, Mark has been tireless in organizing running and walking events that raise money for multiple sclerosis research, as well as provide education to the community about the illness. His enthusiasm is contagious. He has received several community awards for his work. What kind of story did Mark create? He has translated his MS into an inspiring story of courage and dedication to the mission of the MS society. He has integrated his love of challenge and his enthusiasm for life into his ICI story. His illness has lent his story depth and meaning.

AIDS has been a tragic story for society. It is a mortal illness that our society at large has made a tale of God's vengeance. In this atmosphere, the worst thing about testing HIV positive when one is asymptomatic is the social stigma. It is terrifying.

Audrey had been married six months when she and her husband, both attractive and successful New York lawyers, decided to leave their law firms and form a firm of their own. They had to obtain new health insurance. In fulfilling the requirements for application for the health insurance they had to take blood tests. The letter that came from the insurance company changed their lives. Audrey tested positive for HIV. The diagnosis was confirmed. From being two vibrantly happy, successful young people in love and in charge of their lives, Audrey and her husband, Joel, were crushed. They were overwhelmed with fear but they did have each other to talk to. However, there were few, very few other people with whom they could share their feelings. The isolation and the fear of being discovered was sometimes overwhelming, especially for Audrey. She dealt with bouts of disorientation, lost a great deal of interest in her work and felt depressed. Eventually, they asked us for help.

Audrey and Joel each knew that the other had been involved in a number of sexual relationships before they married. The issue for them was not ultimately one of recrimination and guilt. The issue was whether they could overcome feelings of hopelessness and dread, whether they could choose to live with her condition as well as with a chronic illness that needed to be "treated" by a life lived in a healthy, positive, life-affirming way, whether she could trust Joel's love and commitment, and whether she could love him in return.

Having tested HIV positive has become for Audrey and Joel a story of terrible challenge to them to love one another "for better or worse, in sickness and in health." When only four months earlier their love and confidence were enabling them to form their own law firm, now they have to choose one another all over again and choose life itself. They have chosen not to reveal the situation to their families, a decision that has saddened them in its revelation of their lack of trust in some of their family members; at the same time it has made them more dependent upon one another. Joel has become more solicitous of Audrey's needs. Audrey has learned that she must avoid getting tired, that she must eat sensibly and sleep on schedule. She has started to play golf again, has learned exercises that relax her, and takes time to rest. They know now that they will not have children—another awareness that, while it saddens them, can make them more appreciative of their need for one another.

For this young couple, the HIV diagnosis is not a story of shame and punishment at all. It is a story of courageous response to a major life challenge. It is a story of love having to mature quickly, of plans having to be revised, of life having to be lived in a way that makes the present moment and life itself terribly precious.

ICI can be an event in our lives that shapes our narratives toward a peaceful, courageous way of living. It can also be an event that comes to dominate our lives and to suck away the joy in living. Maria was first afflicted with vaginal infections, painful bladder, and terrible menstrual cramps in her early teens. By the time she was diagnosed with endometriosis three years later, Maria had developed a fetish for cleanliness. She bathed several times a day and shampooed her hair so frequently that her body grew raw from scrubbing and her hair became dry and lifeless. She washed her clothes even if she had only tried on an outfit. All food had to be washed before being refrigerated and washed again before she would eat it. She had stopped eating in restaurants, which made dating a tense and awkward situation. When she fell in love with George, whom she considered marrying, arguments about sex strained their relationship. Sex was painful and she would maneuver the time spent with George in such a way as to avoid physical intimacy. Finally, the relationship collapsed in a storm of accusations and bitterness. Antiseptic cleanliness became Maria's futile, sad, and lonely goal. For her, endometriosis is dirty, as is everything else, including sex and Maria herself.

For some individuals, invisible chronic illness is an event, an ongoing event that has been accepted and integrated into their revised life story. Mandie is not a Broadway star but she realizes that her need to be special and her need for attention can be met on a different stage. Mark's life story of optimism and love of activity has been deepened by his illness to become in addition a story of mission and purpose.

In the next chapter we turn to the necessary task of discovering our stories and of testing them to see whether they are true to reality, whether they give us hope and peace, or whether they limit who we are and distort who we might be.

14

Identifying Your Story

Who am I? They . . . tell me
I bore the days of misfortune
equably, smilingly, proudly, like one
    accustomed to win.
Am I then really that which other men tell of?
Or am I only what I myself know of myself?
Restless and longing and sick, like a bird in a
    cage.

Dietrich Bonhoeffer

The story that you live needs to be brought into consciousness. It has enormous power in giving your life direction and meaning. It defines your values and shapes your view of yourself and of your world. Being aware of your story can help to free you from any limitations that it imposes and any untruths that it inflicts. Consciousness of your story can free you to understand yourself more deeply and to change in directions that make your life more livable. As Sam Keen puts it, "You have to take the unconscious myth to get to the conscious autobiography."[1]

How then do you begin to surface your particular narrative? A story has to be told. In telling it, you can begin to understand it more clearly. Sometimes a therapist is the listener. We usually begin a first therapy session by asking the client, "What brings you here?" or by saying something like, "Tell me what's happening." The client then begins to tell his story. His story is not a chronological narrative. He seldom begins, "I was born in Atlanta, Georgia, on November the 3rd, 1946." Rather, he starts to tell about himself in terms of what matters to him. "I'm a professional actor and I have three children. Recently things have been coming apart." Or, "I don't know for sure why I'm here. I'm usually on top of things, but I seem to be losing control. My wife is threatening to leave me unless I get some help. She thinks I drink too much." Or, "Where do I begin? I don't think I love my husband. He's a good man, but I've lost interest. I hate the East. I hate our house. I think I hate my life. I've got to do something."

These opening lines are the beginning of stories. Gradually the client fills out more details of what he values, how he views himself, what his hopes and ambitions are, how his needs are met or not met and how he views his particular problem. Bit by bit the client's story comes into focus. It becomes clear that he identifies very strongly with his career or that he values control or that he attributes his problems to hers or that he is rebelling against the constraints of his lifestyle. Patterns of thought and behavior are identified. Self-image is clarified. Etiology or background causes of the ways that the client thinks, believes, and acts are established. Roles that the client plays or avoids are identified. Scripts that the client lives become clear.

Therapy can be an effective way of uncovering your story, so can participation in workshops devoted to personal narratives. But not everyone chooses this route to self-knowledge. Ask yourself now the following questions to bring to awareness the story and stories that you live by.

Who are your heroes?
What do you think is important in life?
What do you most value?
What does death mean to you?
What does sex mean to you?
What does your work mean to you?
What does God mean to you?
What role did you play in your family?
How would you start to tell someone who you are?

Who are and have been your heroes? You can tell a person by the books he reads. You can also tell him by whom he admires. If Paul told you that Ben Hogan was his childhood hero, you would probably recognize his love of golf. You might also appreciate his having a hero who was, like him, "bantam" and might see his admiration of someone triumphing over adversity. His early hero pointed to an early story. He wanted to be outstanding, even famous. Having had a traumatic birth, and sickly with allergies and colds as a child, Paul was determined to overcome obstacles to success. Other heros for Paul included the self-denying Irish "saint," Matt Talbot, singers from Frank Sinatra to Mario Lanza, and later Bobby Kennedy. Each hero called to a different dimension of Paul and was a role model for another version of his developing story.

A bright successful client with a tendency to melancholy and negative thinking recently identified his father as his hero. As he narrated the memories he had, the father emerged as a good, self-sacrificing family man who had been treated unfairly by life in the person of a weak, complaining wife and by undeserved career mishaps. The client had little trouble seeing how his own story, which demanded hard work but predicted eventual and inevitable unfair treatment, not only sapped the joy from his life and the satisfaction from his achievements but had also become self-fulfilling and self-destructive. It is important to know who we have as heroes if we are to know ourselves and the role models and images we live by.

What is important to you and what do you value? How do your answers to these questions influence your life story? If you have answered, "being loved," how does your life reflect this need to be loved? How does this value affect the way you live? If you wrote, "being happy," how is your life shaped by this desire? If you wrote, "being successful," how is your life organized and directed to meet this goal? Would someone looking at your life have an easy time identifying what is important to you and what it is that you most value? Do you live congruently with your values?

What does death mean to you? Does death mean the end of everything to you? The end of all opportunity? Is it something to be feared? Is it a tragic end or a new beginning? Is it a reunion with those you have loved? Is it an entrance into joy and fulfillment? Does your view of death affect your story?

What does sex mean to you? Is it something natural to be enjoyed? Is it sinful or stressful or dirty? Is it for love, for fun, for children, for control? How does sex fit into your story? For an attractive, thirty-year-old lawyer, Jeanne, sex was a painful area of her life controlled by abstention. Jeanne had received the message in her family that sex was dirty and sinful. In reaction to this attitude, Jeanne rebelled with promiscuous behavior in high school and college, triggering her family's disdain and her own self-hatred. After two abortions, Jeanne determined to avoid sex and to channel her energies into her career. Jeanne's story will be sad and lonely until she gives sex new meaning.

What does your work mean to you? Is your work what you have to do to earn money to play? Is it what gives your life meaning or satisfaction? What role does your work play in your life story? Monica is a thin, nervous woman who came to us as a result of recurring anxiety attacks. She had stopped working to have her baby. The adorable little boy was fifteen months old, but Monica still felt guilty that she no longer worked at her job. In her first two sessions she mentioned twice that she had been making $70,000 a year as a vice president in an insurance company. When confronted about the significance of stating the size of her salary, Monica described her sense of worth and power in earning such an income—a worth and value reinforced by her husband, who had been delighted with the money that she earned and was angry at her refusal to return to work. Monica's job had given her value in society's eyes and in her husband's. Loss of the job threatened her own sense of worth and the esteem that she had experienced from her husband.

What does God mean to you? Does God fit into your story? How? Does God reward you? Punish you? Love you? Is God central or peripheral or nonexistent in your story? God plays a central role in the story of Philip, a fifty-year-old journalist who, despite his chronic fatigue, is active in his church and in charitable activities. His wife of twelve years died after a horrible ordeal with cancer. Philip told us her story.

> When Annie died I wanted to die, too. I knew that the children needed me, but even then I was battling fatigue and loneliness that I can't begin to describe. I think I went for a year with almost no sleep—the nights were the worst. But two years after Annie died, I went to mass by myself one morning. It was a weekday and there was almost no one in church but the priest and me. Suddenly, I had a profound sense of God's presence and a feeling that I was not alone. God seemed to say, "Philip, I'm with you and will be with you. You're not alone." Since then God has been central in my life. I like to think that Annie asked God to give me a break.

What role do you play in your family? Were you the oldest of your family? The baby? The middle child? Were you the beauty? The brain? The good one? The bad one? Were you the responsible one, the rebel, the peacemaker? How has your role in the family influenced your story and the role that you play now?

How would you start to tell someone who you are? Would you start your story by telling about your job? Your childhood? Your parents? (Which one first?) Would you start with, "I'm married," "I'm Jewish," or "I'm forty"? How you begin your story can be indicative of what you think is most important about yourself.

One client began her response to our invitation to tell us about herself with these words,

What is there to tell? It's pretty boring. I don't work. I have four very good kids. I don't know how I deserve them. My husband is a very successful lawyer.

Her opening words reveal a lack of self-worth and confidence. She thinks she and her story are of no interest to anyone. She immediately states that she does not work, probably revealing an attitude that only a career gives life value. She is not worthy of her children. In contrast to her lack of value, her husband is described as "very successful."

Sam Keen, who has written on personal narratives,[2] suggests that we draw a floor plan of the house that we were raised in and then start telling someone what rooms and memories come to mind. He also tells participants at his workshops to imagine that their biography was being printed and that the publisher wants to include ten photographs of them at different times of their lives. What photos would you imagine to be most significant? How true is the story?

Stories are powerful; the less examined they are, the more powerful. If in the story of your illness, you play the role of the bad person who in some way is responsible for being ill, that role will defeat you with guilt and shame. No one will be able to save or console you until you see the story as false and your role in the untrue story as hopeless. If your script has you in the role of the sensible engineer when your real talents lie in photography and artistic achievement, then your depression is probably due to playing the wrong role rather than to chemical imbalance.

Possibly the most important result of inquiry into our stories is that we grow in humility, realizing that we are not holders of the truth but simply narrators of stories that attempt to give meaning to the vast assortment of events that fill our lives.

Central to the task of clarifying your story is externalizing it. This is done by separating yourself from the event that is the present problem. In the example in the preceding chapter concerning Maria and her identification with endometriosis, Maria needs to separate her illness from herself, to externalize it and then begin to have control over it instead of being totally controlled by it. The endometriosis is an illness, a separate, definable malady that unfortunately afflicts a great number of women. It has no connection to cleanliness or lack of it.

Maria can begin to accomplish this externalization by asking herself how the illness affects her life and her relationships. How has it exercised a tyrannical hold on her life? What does she have to learn to break its grip? She has to recognize that the role she has given her symptoms is affecting her marriage and the way she is raising her children. It has caused her to withdraw from her husband and to instill resentment in her children. By beginning to look at the illness as separate from herself, she has begun to take hold of her life again.

As Maria externalizes her illness, she begins to create a new story more congruent with her values as wife and mother, more true to the reality of the illness, more conducive of self-respect and peace. As White and Epson write in *Narrative Means to Therapeutic Ends,* "Through the process of externalization, persons gain a reflexive perspective on their lives, and new options become available to them in challenging the 'truths' that they experience as defining and specifying of them and their relationships."[3]

Ask yourself how your illness is affecting your life and your relationships. Does it determine the view that you have of yourself? Does it decide whether you are attractive or not? Good or bad? Successful or unsuccessful? Does it make you a failure? Does it make you unlovable? Unappealing? Uninteresting? Does it stop you from enjoying, achieving, or loving? How does it affect your relationships? With your friends? With your spouse? With men? With women? With co-workers?

Joan has irritable bowel syndrome. Answering the above questions, she realized that she was allowing her illness to write a very sad story. She viewed herself as a failure for having the illness and for failing to find a cure. Her irritable bowel syndrome led her to view herself as weak, unattractive, and essentially bad. It made her an unappealing, rather boring wife and friend. Her constant quest for cure made enjoyment and celebration of life impossible.

Joan's story ignored the truth of her integrity and intelligence. It did not acknowledge her enormous skill and love as a mother of three small children. It failed to recognize her goodness, compassion, and generosity. As Joan has begun to separate herself from IBS, she has begun to appreciate who she really is and to see her illness simply as what it is. She has opened up more to her husband and expects more real sharing from him. She admits now to friends that she would love to play tennis or go to the theater but might have to back out if she is not well. By externalizing her illness she can admit to others that she has an illness and can realize within herself that *she* has *it* under control rather than the other way around. Your are responsible for making your story a true one. Your illness is yours—you need not be its.

15

Getting and Keeping the Attention of the Health-Care System

My ideal doctor would be my Virgil, leading me through my purgatory or inferno, pointing out the sights as we go. He would resemble Oliver Sacks, the neurologist who wrote *Awakenings* and *The Man Who Mistook His Wife for a Hat*. I can imagine Dr. Sacks entering my condition, looking around at it from the inside like a benevolent landlord with a tenant, trying to see how he could make the premises more livable for me. He would mingle his daemon with mine; we would wrestle with my fate together. Inside every patient, there's a poet trying to get out. My ideal doctor would "read" poetry, my literature. He would see that my sickness has purified me, weakening my worst parts and strengthening the best.

Anatole Broyard

No matter how well you apply your own resources to coping with ICI, you need the help of doctors. Getting this help in a consistently satisfying manner is as essential as it is challenging. You will need perseverance, courage, and skill. You will need to understand your needs and to be committed to getting them met. As is usually the case in getting your needs met by another, a good place to start is by learning to meet the other's needs.

The Patient's Failure to Communicate Effectively

ICI patients often fail to present themselves clearly to their doctors. Clients have revealed to us numerous reasons why their communications with their doctors are frustrating. Some are stymied by fear and feelings of intimidation. Since many patients suffering from invisible illness are women, they may fear prejudice or authoritarian attitudes on the part of male doctors. Patients usually do not think or express themselves clearly when they feel inferior or afraid. Some fear that they are viewed with suspicion, seen as hysterical or as creating symptoms out of stress or depression. Consequently, they edit their complaints or deny them altogether. As one client told us, "I just don't tell him anything that could sound like depression."

Patients tend to view doctors from one of two opposite angles, neither of which facilitates satisfying interaction: with awe for the omniscient father/mother figure; or with distrust for the one who will judge her, charge her, and leave her in no better place than she was before seeing him. Patients with the former view expect too much. They often become disappointed, disillusioned, and angry. Patients with the latter view expect too little. They frequently neglect to make appointments with doctors or are reserved or belligerent in a manner that results in interactions that reinforce their previous attitudes.

What Your Doctor Wants from You

Every day we hear clients' stories of their encounters with doctors. Plus, we have our own stories with either sad or happy endings. We wanted to hear doctors' stories of their experience in treating patients with ICI. A number of clients suggested names of doctors—general practitioners, specialists of all kinds, men and women. Our list was admittedly a select sample of the medical world, but we were deeply impressed by the generosity of the physicians' response. In answer to our question as to the challenges they face in seeing someone with ICI symptoms, four areas of difficulty were mentioned over and over by these medical doctors in separate interviews.

Conflicting agendas. "My task," a ruddy-faced specialist told us, "is to check for every possible medical reason that could explain these symptoms. To accomplish this, I ask a lot of questions. But the patient has her own agenda, which keeps her from answering my questions. For example, if I ask, 'Do you feel the fatigue during exercise or at rest?' She might answer, 'I exercise very sensibly and always have.' I might ask the question four or five times and still not get a clear answer. Her agenda might be to show me that she's not crazy, or that she is not causing her fatigue, or that she's a good girl, or whatever. But my goal of getting necessary information to make a diagnosis is thwarted."

Mind sets. A delightful young general practitioner showed us a recent cover of *Medical World News*. The cover portrayed in cartoon form three people waiting in a doctor's office: a buttoned-up businessman looking at his watch; a fierce-looking woman holding a *Physician's Desk Reference* in her lap; and a little round lady with a box of medicine bottles resting on her lap. He used the cartoon to discuss the mind sets he faces daily. The businessman looking at his watch is saying that the doctor is wasting his valuable time. His manner says, "Do your job quickly and get me back to the real world, where I make my living." The hostile-looking woman is ready for battle and the doctor is the designated enemy. The walking pharmacy is ready to talk endlessly of ailments and cures. The genial doctor pointed out that these are just three of the mind sets that make his work difficult. He added that he could describe many more.

Information overload. A good doctor wants to get to the bottom of a patient's complaint, identify it, understand it, and treat it. But sometimes a patient can so overwhelm him with data that he hardly knows where to begin, proceed, or end.

A woman with ICI might call for an appointment with a complaint about a strange numbness in her legs. The doctor begins the examination with certain expectations about the particular issue for this appointment. He will examine the patient's legs and ask her when, where, and how long she has felt the numbness. He anticipates that the appointment will take a certain period of time. But before he has completed his evaluation, the woman starts telling him about an ongoing headache and about a peculiar tingling in her arms— symptoms that all seem new, strange, and possibly connected. At this point, the physician may begin to feel *information overload*. Each of the patient's complaints is a source of concern for the patient. And now that she has the physician's attention, she wants to let him know all that she has been suffering. The doctor, however, must attend to each complaint individually, even though he may eventually conclude that the complaints are symptomatic of one illness.

He may feel like he's being bombarded with a multitude of physical complaints—possibly connected, possibly not. The appointment is taking longer than he anticipated and he knows that other patients are waiting. He is overloaded with data that he lacks time to process. He knows that he cannot satisfy himself or the patient. By the way, the businessman with the watch is probably his next patient.

Lack of clarity. All the doctors we spoke with, general practitioners and specialists alike, complained that getting clear, precise information from the patient was their biggest challenge. These doctors told stories of imprecise, inaccurate accounts of symptoms. They talked of patient exaggeration, denial, and forgetfulness. Doctors need patients to listen to their questions, to be clear and succinct in their reporting of symptoms, and to be understanding of the doctor's difficult task. Mutual understanding between patient and doctor is the desired goal. ICI threatens such understanding.

Doctor–Patient Relationship

As we discussed in Chapter 7, the unmeasurable nature of invisible chronic illness can precipitate lack of understanding by the scientifically oriented doctor—a lack that can degenerate into impatience, distrust, and suspicion. We tend not to treat kindly what we don't understand, and perplexed doctors can unwittingly be quite cruel. On the other hand, self-doubting, vulnerable ICI patients can be so unclear in relating their symptoms as to trigger the very impatience and suspicion that they fear. An interchange between Catherine, who suffers from "mild" MS, and her neurologist demonstrates the complexity of what might seem a simple interaction. Catherine is a registered psychiatric nurse. Prior to the appointment with her neurologist, Catherine had been experiencing frightening and embarrassing mental problems. While talking to a patient, Catherine might have been saying, "There are several points involved here," and then go blank after stating the first point. Her brain seemed to have lost its capacity to hold information while other information was being relayed. During the appointment Catherine started to narrate these troubling events. Before she could describe her feelings of fear, the neurologist stated flatly, "Multiple sclerosis does not impair mental functioning," and then turned his attention to Catherine's magnetic resonance imaging results.

Catherine was baffled. With personal and professional interest she had read extensive medical journal articles on MS. A number of these articles had discussed in great detail the often bizarre forms of cognitive impairment due to multiple sclerosis. Catherine, who trusts her neurologist's competence, was left with a jumbled assortment of feelings and speculations. She considered refuting the doctor's assertion, but such behavior seemed inappropriate. She feared sounding aggressive. Then she thought that the neurologist surely must know more than she about MS, so perhaps the doctor was trying to reassure her to keep her from worrying. At the same time, Catherine felt angry at being dismissed in her description of such troubling symptoms. In her vulnerability, she began to doubt herself: Maybe she *was* imagining the experiences, or exaggerating them, or even causing them out of fear. Yet, the incidents had surely happened. If they were not due to MS, was something else seriously wrong with her? Or was she indeed losing her mind? None of these thoughts or feelings was shared with the doctor. Some of her confidence in the doctor had been shaken; her rather fragile inner peace had been shaken even more. She dreaded the inevitable question she would face at home, "What did the doctor say?"

Patients need the doctor to be caring and patient, attentive and thorough. At the same time, patients need to regard doctors realistically as fellow adults who can bring training and insight to bear on their problems to the degree that the patients make themselves as clear as possible. Awe and distrust are not feelings conducive to effective interaction.

Patients with a realistic understanding of the doctor and his role will not look for omniscience or even for fatherly or motherly care. They will attempt to understand his busy schedule and so will be prepared to discuss their symptoms as clearly and concisely as possible. Doctors have told us the strain that patients put on their patience by not coming to the point, by not remembering important details, or by going on at length about issues that are not pertinent. We advise clients to keep accurate records of their symptoms, noting the kind of symptoms, intensity, duration, and precipitating factors and to have this record with them when visiting their doctor. It is important, despite feelings of vulnerability and self-doubt, for the patient to present himself as clearly and confidently as possible, treating the doctor with respect, not awe, and with trust, not fear and distrust.

The Doctor and His Feelings

Renowned psychologist Carl Rogers once remarked: "I seldom say anything negative or angry to a patient. My role makes me too powerful. A sharp remark from me in my role of Father-Authority-Doctor can sound like a clap of thunder."[1]

Surrounded by the trappings of power and position, doctors can easily lose awareness of the patient's vulnerability. While we do not suggest that doctors never reveal their feelings, we do urge them to be very aware of the impact of their words on their patients. Doctors need to put their imagination to work to achieve genuine understanding of the patients' perspective. Periodically, it would be illuminating for doctors to imagine themselves half-robed, ill, needy, dependent, and on the receiving end of thermometers, proddings, questions, admonitions, and advice. Then doctors might empathize more deeply with their patients' feelings of confusion, helplessness, and fear. Like the physician played by William Hurt in the movie, *The Doctor,* they need to confront their own weakness and vulnerability. Imbued with such understanding, the doctor would be moved to listen, to admit not knowing, to be tender and humble. Salinger, in his novel, *Franny and Zooey,* has Zooey say regarding his confused sister, Franny, that he'd send her to a psychiatrist, but "He'd have to believe that it's through the grace of God that he has the native intelligence to be able to help his goddam patients at all."[2] Doctors confronted with invisible illness need saintly qualities to be effective in their godly work.

Doctors need to pursue awareness of their own feelings, needs, and prejudices. When the neurologist stated categorically that MS does not affect cognitive functioning, was he aware of what his feeling was at that moment? For example, he might have been *concerned* that Catherine was panic-stricken and hoped to reassure her, or he might have been *impatient* that Catherine was introducing more symptoms that were nonmeasurable, or *suspicious* of Catherine, or *threatened* by her professional knowledge. Whatever the feeling, that feeling prompted his statement.

Feelings have an immediate influence on our behavior. For example, if I am afraid of meeting someone, I might very well act in a way to avoid the meeting. I might "forget" the party at which I was to be present, or get ill that day, or arrange a business meeting that prevents me from being present. In this case, my feeling is *governing* my behavior. However, if I admit that feeling to myself, I can then say, "Hold on now; okay, I'm afraid. How do I want to act?" At that point, I am in a position to act more freely and responsibly. I do not deny the feeling, nor does it control me. In the previous example, if the neurologist were feeling impatient with Catherine, he would simply need to "hold it," in order to gain control of himself. He might do the proverbial "count to ten" and then choose to listen more intently to Catherine's experience of this symptom and to her feelings of fear being generated by it. He might choose to ask Catherine questions about the symptoms, being careful not to do so impatiently. He might sensitively share with Catherine his feelings of concern that Catherine might be reacting too strongly to the symptom and remind her that she has overreacted to earlier symptoms. He might even need to leave the examining room for a few minutes to settle his impatience and remain nonjudgmental and professional.

None of these choices is possible if the doctor is not aware of his feelings. Our experience is that doctors, like most people, are not sufficiently aware of their feelings to avoid being controlled by them. Being so aware demands focus and attention. Most of us can answer the question, "What are you thinking?" The question as to what we are feeling leaves us blank. We usually don't know what we are feeling unless the feeling is quite strong, and even then we confuse anger with hurt and frustration with loneliness. Doctors need to listen to their feelings throughout the day and be willing to admit them to themselves.

To admit feelings demands humility and self-knowledge, especially to acknowledge feelings that do not seem to fit one's self-image or role. For example, feelings of confusion or fear or inferiority might be totally unacceptable to the doctor's view of himself; therefore, they might be blocked from awareness or denied—so might feelings of sexual attraction, hurt, or anger. Such denial is not conscious. It stems from role-playing. Yet such lack of authentic, humble self-awareness is a serious impediment to effective meeting. If the doctor is not genuinely in tune with meeting himself, he has little chance of effectively meeting his patient.

The doctor must be aware also of needs and prejudices if he is to relate freely and responsibly with patients. Some doctors need to appear all-knowing. They state opinions as facts and possibilities as certainties. Some need to be right and can't admit mistakes or tolerate any challenge to their authority. Prejudice blinds doctors as it does all of us. Many male doctors maintain negative attitudes toward women. The same complaint that can elicit sympathy and interest when made by a male patient can prompt impatience and even derision when coming from a woman. Premenstrual syndrome (PMS), for example, can produce a multitude of symptoms; many doctors may react by dismissing most complaints. Doctors must demand of themselves growth in self-knowledge and training in skills of communication.

What Do You Want from Your Doctor?

Anatole Broyard, the former editor of the *New York Times Book Review*, wrote an article in the *New York Times Magazine* on what he hoped for from a doctor. He was dying from cancer and had firsthand experience with an array of physicians. He titled his article, "Doctor, Talk to Me." Many patients would add, "And Listen to Me."

Ask yourself what you want from your doctor and then, when you have established your needs, be determined to get them met. Most patients with invisible chronic illnesses talk of wanting to be met in a genuine, understanding way. Sandy, an articulate fifty-year-old writer who suffers with fibromyalgia, probably spoke for all patients when she expressed her needs in a doctor,

> I want the doctor to be present to me in an undistracted, alert, and friendly manner. I desire a combination of

warmth and competence. I need to trust that I matter to the doctor, that he knows me, cares for me, respects me, and trusts me. I need the sense that he has truly reflected on my illness and tried to understand how specifically the illness affects my life. The illness is unique to me, I need to feel that it is not routine to him.

Thomas L. English, M.D., suffers from chronic fatigue syndrome. In an article he wrote in a medical journal, he states, "I have survived because of caring friends and fellow patients and because of a few committed physicians who kept their mind open. They truly listened. They thought long and hard. Many were and still are ridiculed for taking CFS seriously."[3]

Doctors are cautioned in their training to avoid emotional involvement with patients and to maintain professional distance. In our age of malpractice suits, such distance can seem all the more necessary. But necessary detachment can degenerate into aloofness. Self-protective fear of the patient makes healing contact highly unlikely. Doctors, like all of us, need to learn how to meet in a manner that evokes trust. Without this trust, the patient is not safe to share openly all that she needs to discuss. Often what she needs to share seems embarrassing, shameful. She has to know that in her doctor she has a wise, honest, trustworthy person in whom she can confide. A young neurologist who has endeared herself to some of our clients told us how heavy she feels after having to give a serious diagnosis to a patient. This lovely young woman touches her patients because she lets them touch her.

Doctors who instill trust in our clients are treasured. A very sensitive client who hides behind a hard-boiled, tough-talking shield told us what it was like to find a doctor she trusts.

I came home from my first visit and cried. Me! He came out into the waiting room to meet me and looked me right in the face. Ordinarily I would have thought, my

God, what's this, but I felt immediate trust. He's got no bullshit. He's direct. He's got a sense of humor. He didn't rush me. And he listened. I felt like my search was over— I guess that's why I cried.

If you have an invisible chronic illness, you are likely to visit several doctors. Don't settle for one with whom you are not comfortable, one to whom you cannot talk, one who does not listen. Broyard writes, "Every patient invites the doctor to combine the role of priest, the philosopher, the poet, the scholar."[4] Your needs are very significant, and it will take a special physician to meet them. But, thank God, profoundly beautiful men and women serve as doctors. Ask friends, consult associations serving your illness, ask a priest, rabbi, or minister whom you trust.

Doctors of such human distinction are a godsend to their patients. But by growing in all their human capabilities, especially their ability to instill trust by communicating effectively, doctors breathe new life into their own healing careers. Broyard wrote with the conviction of one who is dying,

> Not every patient can be saved, but his illness may be eased by the way the doctor responds to him—and in responding to him, the doctor may save himself. But first he must become a student again; he has to dissect the cadaver of his professional persona; he must see that his silence and neutrality are unnatural. It may be necessary to give up some of his authority in exchange for his humanity, but as the old family doctors knew, this is not a bad bargain. In learning to talk to his patients, the doctor may talk himself back into loving his work. He has little to lose and much to gain by letting the sick man into his heart. If he does, they can share, as few others can, the wonder, terror, and exaltation of being on the edge of being, between the natural and the supernatural.[5]

16

Coping with ICI in the Family

> To storm a breach, conduct an embassy, govern a people, these are brilliant actions; to scold, to laugh . . . and deal gently and justly with one's family and oneself . . . that is something more rare, more difficult, and less noticed in the world.
>
> *Montaigne*

Almost every person with ICI needs the support and understanding of her family—spouses, parents, siblings, children. Nowhere in her life is good communication needed more. It is here that her needs are most pronounced. Many of her needs and those of her family members are so profound and personal that the feelings they generate can be of shattering intensity. Unfortunately, invisible chronic illness provokes tremendous family tension and so strains relationships that among sufferers divorce is common. Where effective communication is so desperately needed, it is frequently absent.

Certainly, no loving family member intentionally refuses to communicate. Yet most of us, whether ill or not, are frequently frustrated by a spouse, a child, or a parent whom we perceive as not being open or as not listening. Family members who want to be a source of comfort to the one who is ill unintentionally neglect listening for the seemingly easier offerings of "comforting" words and such advice as "Don't worry," "Try to think positively," "Things could be worse."

The person with ICI is often overwhelmed with feelings. She needs to be able to identify these feelings and to share them with the people in her life who matter most. Her family members have a similar need. Unfortunately, most individuals with ICI and most people in general don't know how to share their feelings directly. Instead they act out their feelings through some form of attack or withdrawal. The sad result is that they seldom truly release their feelings and even less frequently experience understanding.

Ted's wife, Winnie, was diagnosed with ulcerative colitis over a year ago. He came with her to consult us regarding their communication impasse. He told the story from his viewpoint.

> I come home from work not knowing what the hell to expect. One day Winnie will be hell on wheels—bitchy, complaining, you know, like there's no way of getting near her. Another day she'll either be in bed or might as well be. She won't talk, will hardly let on that I've gotten home. I don't know what's eating her, but I can't take much more.

Winnie's response was almost predictable. For every spouse who doesn't talk, there is usually a spouse who doesn't listen.

> I'd love to tell you how I feel. But every time I've tried, you've cut me off. If I'm angry about feeling so lousy, you look at me like I'm a bitch. If I'm sad, you say I'm feeling sorry for myself. If I try to say I'm afraid, you say that's crazy. So, hell yes, I'm angry and don't talk. I don't want to get shot down.

Supportive Spouses

A recent study reported in the *New York Times*[1] confirmed our overwhelming clinical experience. "How spouses treat their partner suffering a chronic illness . . . has a more profound impact than might be expected on how well sick partners mentally adjust to the suffering." The researchers found that mild grumbling or even relatively benign comments had quite damaging results. If a husband was critical of his sick wife, the study found that she developed very negative attitudes toward her illness and spent much time in wishful thinking, hoping that the illness would go away. But when the wife felt that her husband was supportive, she was more likely to adopt attitudes that made the suffering more tolerable. In fact, many of these women developed very positive viewpoints that the illness had become for them a source of growth.

In our experiences, no one is more important to the married person with ICI than her spouse. He is a mirror into which she looks to see herself. Made vulnerable by her illness, she fears that she will see herself as ugly, undesirable, unlovable. Lovely women looking toward their husbands sometimes see themselves as in a funhouse mirror: gross and distorted. But those with husbands who listen, who share themselves openly, and who communicate can begin to see themselves as needed, admired, understood, and loved. They can see themselves as someone who triumphs over adversity instead of one who gives into an imaginary illness. In Shakespeare's words,

> Love is not love which alters
> When it alteration finds.[2]

Robin is a petite, olive-skinned brunette. She has always been considered "the beauty" in her family. Since she has been taking the anti-inflammatory drug prednisone, her face has become puffy and round and her body is somewhat bloated. She described the difficulty of coping with the changes in her appearance and the need she feels for her husband's affirmation.

I hate looking in a mirror, yet I feel compulsive about looking at myself. It's almost like I think I'll get my face back if I keep looking at it. Over and over and over I keep looking to see if the puffiness has disappeared. Thank God for Jim. He doesn't seem to mind. Yet, I know he loves me "pixie faced," as he used to say. He calls me "beautiful" and asks, "How's my beauty?" It probably sounds silly and vain, but I need to hear it.

Jennifer is very thin but her abdomen is frequently distended by her irritable bowel syndrome. There are many days when most of her clothes won't fit at all. But, as she told us,

> Hank is incredible. If I'm still in bed when he leaves for work, he'll leave me notes telling me that he loves me, giving me the weather report, and hoping that I have a good day. To him I seem attractive, even if I feel gross.

Frequently, it is very hard for the chronically ill person to see herself as lovely and loved. It can be frustrating for a husband to find his wife self-doubting and doubting of his love. He needs to understand his wife's difficulty in really trusting his affection and desire for her. He needs to be aware of how hard it can be for her to trust when she is struggling with feelings of fear, vulnerability, and inadequacy. And she needs to appreciate how hurt he can be in being doubted.

No matter how loving and supportive a spouse might be, he has his own feelings and needs, which are deeply affected by his partner's illness. He needs her to trust in him and accept his love and admiration. He needs her, sometimes, not to focus on or talk about her illness. He needs her attention and care. He needs her to be hopeful and optimistic. He needs her to be a companion on walks, going out to dinner, making love, skiing or playing tennis, in any hobby they have enjoyed in the past together. He might need her to bring in an income. When these needs cannot be met, he may feel disappointed, hurt, frustrated, and then guilty for having these feelings. He has to be free to admit these needs and feelings, even at the risk of hurting the one he loves most.

When the feelings are denied, not only do they fester into judgments about his spouse or about himself, but the denial also promotes distrust. Once these needs and feelings are admitted and accepted as natural and understandable, then the couple can be creative in developing new ways of being together, new ways of meeting their individual needs.

Laurie and Todd are only in their thirties, but have been married for fifteen years. They talked about how they have adapted to Laurie's lupus.

Todd: We used to do everything together. We've been together since high school. We both like sports, so we've been tennis partners at this little club we belong to. We like to bowl with friends. We used to go camping with the kids almost every year. Now a lot of the times I have to play tennis with someone else. I didn't play at all for a while, but that wasn't good for either of us.

Laurie: God, that really made me feel guilty. Sometimes I go and watch him play. But we're doing some stuff we've never done before. Like skiing. Todd will ski with the kids in the morning and then we'll have a real nice lunch on the mountain or in town. Then we'll walk around.

Todd: I look forward to the long lunches together. Then maybe I'll make a few runs at the end of the day. Plus, we've started going to the movies and we've even gone to some dinner theaters. What the hell. We've got one another and two great kids.

Laurie: It does seem like we've gotten closer. Don't you think Todd?

Todd: No question. And we were pretty good before.

Husbands and wives need to listen to one another, to risk being totally open to one another, and as Bernard Gunther and Corita Kent said,

To be of love a little more careful
than of anything else.[3]

Other family members are swamped with feelings when
someone they love suffers from ICI. Their needs, frequently not identified or admitted, are that their daughter
or mother be well or, if she is ill, that the disease be diagnosed, treated, and cured. They need also for their lives not
to be disturbed by fear for the health of a loved one, by
having to care for an invalid, or by suffering the loss of an
active companion. They struggle with their suspicions that
the ICI patient may not be genuinely sick, and they dread
the possibility that the patient is terribly ill. These needs and
struggles trigger feelings. For the family member, these
feelings interfere with effective listening. As it is with the
patient, it is very hard for loved ones to listen to the patient
when struggling with their own mixed feelings.

Friends and acquaintances fear invading privacy or are
uncomfortable with descriptions of symptoms or expressions of suffering and fear. They frequently try to keep the
conversation "light" or to avoid any topic that may segue
into a discussion of the patient's illness. Unaware, perhaps,
of their own feelings of disgust, embarrassment, suspicion,
distrust, or fear for the patient's well-being, friends may
avoid the topic of illness completely. The effect of the
avoidance is to deprive the patient of an opportunity to talk
and to be heard. It also deprives the patient of the opportunity to listen and come to understand the friend more deeply.
Admittedly, it is not easy to share feelings of distrust, for
example, nor are they easy to hear.

Roger, a senior in high school who suffers with an
inflammatory bowel disease, came to us with his mother
and father. They appeared to be uncomfortable and admitted that the three of them had never sat together to talk.
Roger remarked, "We've had discussions, of course, about
when I failed a subject or about what the latest doctor had
said, but they, my parents, have never talked to me about
what is happening to me." His parents looked surprised as

he spoke. His father responded quickly, saying, "Of course we have, Roger, we talk all the time. We talked last night." Roger retorted, "No, you talked. You didn't hear a thing I said." Neither Roger nor his father was sharing what was happening within as he spoke, nor did they listen to each other. Roger's father looked frustrated and turned away. Then he looked back at Roger and said, "Roger, I really don't know what to say to you. I regret that you don't think I want to know what it's been like for you feeling sick all these years. But sometimes it's hard to talk to you. You seem like you're angry all the time. I never know if you're angry at us or if you're feeling sick." Roger glared at his father; when asked if he heard what his father was feeling, he said, "Yeah, I know, he thinks I'm always grouchy."

Roger failed to hear his father's feelings and did what most of us tend to do. Instead of hearing his father's feelings, he heard his father making a judgment about him—"You're grouchy." A frequent failure in listening is the tendency to search in someone's disclosure for "What are you saying about me?" Listening demands that you place your own concerns and feelings on hold in order to place yourself in the shoes of the other person, to be empathic and hear *only* what the person is saying about *himself.* Roger heard his father's judgment about him—"grouchy." Even if he had heard his father's perceptions: "You seem angry all the time. I never know if you're angry at us or you're feeling sick," he would have heard words only *about himself* and how he appeared.

The task for Roger and for all of us is to hear what the speaker is feeling and needing when he perceives certain behaviors. In this case, Roger would have heard his father's vulnerability, his fear that his son would pounce on him in anger, as well as his confusion regarding Roger's moods and physical condition. Roger admitted later that he felt very vulnerable, in general. He believed that most people did not trust that he was genuinely sick. He feared that his father, most of all, didn't trust him and viewed him generally as a crybaby and as grouchy. In his vulnerability and fear of his father's perception of him, he was ready to hear his father call him grouchy. He had little room to hear his father's feeling of regret and tentativeness in approaching Roger.

Another pitfall that undermines real listening is the tendency to hear an attack in the person's disclosure of feelings. Typically, when we think we are being attacked, we defend. One patient who has endometriosis, for example, shared with her husband that she was afraid that sex was so painful sometimes that she felt like making love less and less. Her husband retorted, "I never forced you to make love." When he took some time to reflect on why he had reacted with these words, he commented, "I suppose the truth is I have never really felt sure that Brenda likes sex with me. I have always had a suspicion that she thinks I make her make love whenever I want it." His feelings of doubt and suspicion kept him from hearing Brenda's fear of the pain in sex.

Ironically, listening is impeded at times by love and care. When a patient feels discouraged, frightened, or hopeless, it is exceedingly challenging for someone who loves the patient to hear the feelings without wanting to "fix" the problem. The tendency of the family member, partner, or friend is to offer advice and try to solve the problem. Where invisible chronic illnesses are concerned, few if any of the inherent "problems" can be solved. No one can take pain or fatigue away, no one can cure a chronic illness, no one can force a diagnosis to be made, and no one can produce the perfect remedy. When a patient is suffering from pain, discouraged with fatigue, angry at a doctor's insensitivity, frustrated with an insurance company that refuses to pay, or scared of future disability, it is tempting for the person to offer pain relievers, suggest a "new" treatment plan, encourage the patient to take the insurance company to court, or disparage the doctor. To listen deeply to the patient's suffering, discouragement, anger, frustration, and fear, the listener must resist the temptation to solve the problem. Problem-solving most often comes from feelings of helplessness within the listener. It is daunting to face the reality that we cannot take away pain, cure a disease, and protect the one we love.

Facing the myriad difficulties of ICI with someone we love is an awesome responsibility. We are tempted when we hear that someone suffers to take the suffering away. In most instances of life we cannot do so. We can, however, be a profound source of comfort to another person when we listen. The trials of ICI become easier to accept when we trust that by honestly and deeply listening we can provide comfort.

Role Changes

Some of the coping that is required in families with a sick member involves changing roles. We tend to identify with the roles we play, so changing our role can be threatening to our sense of self. If you have been the energetic one who got everything ready for a family vacation, you can feel an awful sense of worthlessness lying on the living room couch with spouse and children bustling around you. If you were the responsible parent—present on school nights, active in parent-teacher committees, on call for school volunteer programs—you can feel anxiety and guilt at not being the all-American parent. If you were the dynamic dad before MS, being the crippled dad can strip away all sense of authority.

Often the role change involves shifting from independence to dependence. Jeanne is a bright young woman, the youngest daughter of loving parents. She has always shown initiative and ambition. She earned her own money all through high school with an assortment of jobs from waitress in a diner to salesgirl at Macy's. After high school, Jeanne attended Katherine Gibbs secretarial school and graduated to a high-paying job. At twenty-two, she had her own small apartment and a car. Three years later fibromyalgia began to undermine her independence. Her mother spent hours with Jeanne, driving her to doctors, helping her clean her apartment, cooking some of her meals. Finally, Jeanne and her parents concluded that it would be easier on all of the family if she moved back into her parents' home. For Jeanne, this move was traumatic.

> I couldn't get used to it. I know that I needed help, but I had never realized how much I needed privacy and the sense of being able to do things when and how I wanted. Now I can't skip a meal or stay out late, let alone over-night. I can't even leave my bed unmade without upset-ting my mother. They worry too much. They know every move I make. It's driving me nuts. I can't have friends over for the evening. I just pray to God I can get strong enough to move out soon. We've been close as a family, but we're gonna be killing each other if this keeps up.

It is not difficult to imagine the tensions experienced by Jeanne's parents. They are having to revert to caretaker roles that they had performed well but had felt relieved to aban-don. The patience they once possessed is strained. The quiet routine that they have been developing has been disturbed. Their other two daughters are making demands for atten-tion and show signs of jealousy.

Whenever one member of a family changes his or her role it puts pressure on others in the family to change. Before chronic fatigue set in, Rhonda had been the energetic center of her family. She had reveled in the role of super-mom, responsible daughter and daughter-in-law, and attractive "proper" wife to her bank vice-president husband. After some soul-searching family conferences, Rhonda was able to report.

> It's different now for all of us. I think we've all had to change. Bob has been sensational. I think I used to shield him from most family responsibility while he focused on work. I even remembered his parents' birthdays. I bought all the gifts for everyone—even his Christmas gift for me. Can you believe that? I was a family travel agent, family bookkeeper, social secretary, cook, chauf-

feur. You name it. The kids did next to nothing at home and Bob did nothing. Now, Sara and Jeff (eleven and thirteen years old) frequently prepare dinner. They do their laundry. Bob checks on them in the morning and sometimes drives them to school. He attended the last parent-teacher conferences and he called his mother last month for her birthday. I'm reading more and have become interested in some church activities that don't demand much effort or my being out at night. We're better as a family now. It hasn't been easy to change, but necessary.

Many of us are resistant to change. We become entrenched in our roles and daily habits. If we are moved to change, there are family members who will resent change and try to dissuade us. "What's wrong with the way you were?" "But you've always done that." "I'll bet this is because of that new support group you joined." Change threatens what people expect of us and also what will be expected of them. "What will happen to the kids?" "What will my friends think?" "What about the company dinner?" "What about my dinner?" It takes courage to admit that we must let go of what we have known. It can take even more courage to resist the pressures of those we love and whom we hate to disappoint.

The Exacerbation-Remission Cycle's Effect on Roles

The continual flux of ICI symptoms from intense suffering to relatively acceptable levels of wellness makes adjusting to family role changes all the more perplexing. Mary Ellen is a thirty-two-year-old mother of two small girls. Three years ago she suffered her first acute exacerbation of MS. Mary Ellen was not hospitalized, but the total exhaustion she experienced forced her to lie down for most of the day. Her husband, who is in business for himself, took over much of the care of their children and Mary Ellen's mother came in daily to help. Two months later, the MS fatigue greatly subsided and, though Mary Ellen still tired easily, she was able to take up most of her former responsibilities. She described what happened next in her journal.

> I had no idea what getting going again would be like. I couldn't wait to be my old self, but I miss the attention of my mother and I miss Terry being around so much and being so caring of me. He is putting more time than ever into the business but says he has to after neglecting it so much in the last couple of months. The kids are spoiled now and are really testing me. I know it will settle down, but I wouldn't mind going back to bed and watching soaps.

When she wrote that entry Mary Ellen had no idea that a year later another exacerbation would put her back in bed and that the process of readjustment would have to be repeated all over again. ICI does not allow for establishing permanently secure ways of living. Mary Ellen and all those with ICI can live only one day at a time, ready to respond to that day with the energy and health they possess. Today, Mary Ellen might be captain; tomorrow, barely able to be crew. Today, commanding active mother; tomorrow, weak and exhausted patient. Those close to her will be likewise challenged to adapt quickly to new responsibilities, new expectations of her and of themselves. ICI does not allow complacency. It constantly, in the face of nonconstancy, demands the maturity to be flexible.

Making Plans

Nowhere is flexibility in the family coping with ICI needed more than when the family makes plans. A July vacation planned in March might have to be scuttled in June just in time to obtain a refund on the deposit. Or the family can keep the reservation and hope for a quick remission. For the person with IBS, accepting a weekend dinner invitation is a gamble. You are probably not aware of how much planning ahead you do in your family until you begin to fear any planning is foolhardy. Planning for a second child when you are not sure how you will be suffering before, during, and after pregnancy can be harrowing.

Planning an addition on the house in time of remission is stymied by images of trying to cope with construction disruption if an exacerbation strikes. Planning a move when feeling well is threatened by thoughts of dependency on doctors and support groups when you are ill. Planning a job change is complicated by concerns about insurance coverage for preexisting conditions.

Carla has IBS. She told us she has learned to cope with invitations.

> I've learned to tell people right away that I'll be happy to accept the invitation but that I have an illness that might cause me to cancel. If that is okay, fine. If it would be too disruptive to them, I understand. It has taken a lot of pressure off me. I was constantly afraid of hurting people by refusing or by canceling. I've gotten natural with it and most people have been really good.

Jenny's lupus makes planning difficult. She listed some of her ways of handling the problem.

> We never make reservations that have a no-refund policy. I always put in writing when making a reservation that I am ill and might be forced to cancel and request a written agreement covering refunds. My doctor has written a letter for me that I have used with airlines to obtain a refund on a canceled flight. We go ahead and plan trips because we need to get away and love to travel. I just take precautions and feel okay if we have to cancel. I don't want to stop living.

Planning your life is necessary; to do so you have to accept your illness and its limitations. You won't be able to plan with the blithe confidence of those who are well. And yet, the unforeseen afflicts all people. If you are self-accepting, patient with yourself, and open with your friends, you can go about the necessary planning that is part of living. To do otherwise would be unfair to yourself and to your friends. It would be giving in to your illness in a way that would eventually make your life not worth living.

Communicating with the Employer

We would like to insert at this point some thoughts about revealing your illness at work. One of the questions we are asked most frequently when addressing groups of ICI patients is "Should I tell my employer about my illness?" An accountant who asked this question after a meeting of the MS Society summed up many common concerns:

> I've been working for an accounting firm for eight years and I'm now coming due to be considered for partner. I'm afraid that if I say anything about having MS, I'll kill my chances. Yet, it seems unfair or dishonest not to tell my boss. Plus, I've had to miss a number of days of work and have a ton of doctor's appointments. I want to explain. But I don't want to be taken off important accounts. One day I decide to tell him, then I decide to wait. What do you think I should do?

The accountant evidently would like to be open about his illness. He wants to be understood regarding his absences and trusted in his commitment. He wants to be fair to his company and especially to his boss. Yet, he fears the consequences of revealing his condition. Each person must respond to his unique situation. You have to balance your fears of the effect of your disclosure with the stress of keeping your illness secret. You need to examine your reluctance to admit your illness. Is distrust of your boss's reaction fully warranted? Is embarrassment motivating your reticence? You need to consider if the effects of the illness on your performance are such that the company has a right to be informed. After considering your needs and rights and those of your employer, hopefully you can make a wise decision. If that decision, in fairness to yourself and to your employer, is to divulge the fact of your illness, then you must be sure to communicate this fact as effectively as possible.

The employer has a right to know as precisely as possible what he can expect from the employee. In what manner will the illness be a handicap? How will it affect performance and to what extent? Will it get worse? The very nature of the chronic illnesses that we are discussing makes exact answers to such questions almost impossible. Yet, it is the ICI sufferer's challenge and responsibility to communicate very clearly regarding these concerns. You need to communicate your understanding and appreciation of the boss's questions. Getting hurt or being defensive or evasive is totally unproductive, helping neither you nor your boss. Rather, you should help him or her understand the illness and its ramifications for your performance as thoroughly as you are able. At the same time you will have to apprise your boss of your own needs, which might include a need for confidentiality. Your boss might feel obliged to inform his superior, but confidentiality can still be preserved. You might want to discuss your need for frequent doctor appointments, for certain working conditions, for possible alterations in your schedule.

Once the decision has been made to reveal the illness at work and to communicate clearly regarding its ramifications, you must be ready to handle the consequences of your revelation. One of the consequences is often solicitude, which can be welcome but also embarrassing. Clients have shared with us their sense of embarrassment at being treated differently from everyone else or from how they were formerly treated. Many voice the awkwardness of being treated like cripples.

Jane works as part of a team that conducts management training seminars. At a recent seminar, chairs, podium, and tables had to be arranged. The team members insisted that Jane be seated while they did the arranging. She was grateful, yet felt isolated and fearful as they laughed and joked as they worked. She also felt weak and helpless and feared that these feelings would influence the team's view of her during the seminar itself. In contrast, we know several invisible chronic illness sufferers who tend to dominate others in order to overcome feelings of weakness. Such behavior is called reaction formation by psychologists and obnoxious by those experiencing it.

The ICI sufferer has to accept the reality of his illness and the limitations that it imposes. He might have to assert the truth of these limitations to a boss or a colleague responsible for negotiating work schedules or making contingency plans for periods of debilitating symptoms. Facing the facts of the illness is essential for clear, satisfying interactions. The more self-accepting and at ease the person who has the ICI, the more others will be at ease in his presence. Bosses and colleagues get their cues from you as to when the illness can be mentioned and what adjustments to it need be made. Telling certain truths in the workplace is often viewed as threatening, if not occupational suicide. But our experience has been that in general employers, bosses, and colleagues respond to trust and to clear communication about the illness with understanding and with appreciation for being informed. Our clients frequently report how moved they have been by the mature and compassionate response of their superiors and peers. Admitting illness at work can eliminate the defensiveness and self-pity that are the consequences of withholding the truth about being ill. Prudent revelation can foster more trust between you and your employers, more relief for you, and more understanding from them.

17

Saying What You Feel

Oh, the comfort
The inexpressible comfort
Of feeling safe with a person
Having neither to weigh thoughts
Nor measure words
But pouring them
All right out, just as they are
Chaff and grain together,
Certain that a faithful hand will
Take and sift them.
And with the breath of kindness
Blow the rest away.

Dinah Craik

The building blocks of effective personal communication are feelings, needs, and perceptions. Feelings come
from needs met or not met. They color our perceptions and
drive our behavior. To communicate honestly and effectively, the speaker needs to be aware of his feelings and the
need from which they spring. He needs to connect the feelings with his perceptions. Finally, he needs to acquire the
skill of stating that feeling and perception without blame or
judgment.

Example #1: Health-Care Provider and Patient

Ann is struggling with fibromyalgia and has been encouraged by her neurologist to see a physical therapist. She com-

plains about her session with him and describes their last conversation.

Ann: These exercises are very difficult. It seems like the harder I try, the more pain I feel.

Therapist: Your muscles are being strengthened by the exercises even though you might be feeling some pain now.

Ann: I know. You told me that last week, but every time I did them this week I had to rest for hours and the pain is worse. I am going to stop doing them now. They hurt too much.

Therapist: You know if you don't try harder and get a better attitude, you will never feel well.

Whatever the therapist's intention in making the statement, "If you don't try harder and get a better attitude, you will never feel well," he primarily sends a message to the patient that implies:

> You don't try hard.
> You don't have a good attitude.
> It is your fault that you don't feel well.
> You may *never* feel well.

If the therapist were questioned, he probably would emphatically deny any intention to direct such discouraging messages to the patient. He might claim that his intent is to motivate. The way he communicates, though, can leave the patient feeling defensive and discouraged—hardly feelings that lead to motivated behavior. To communicate his intention more effectively, the therapist must be more aware of his inner world—his needs and his feelings. Equipped with such awareness, the therapist can be more confident that what he shares is that which he genuinely intends to share. He must ask himself:

What are my needs?

To see the patient improve?

To be an effective therapist?

To work with a "cooperative" patient?

What am I feeling?

Impatience?

Concern?

Fear?

Frustration?

Care?

Feelings are connected intimately to needs. The therapist's need to see the patient progress over the weeks of therapy or to hear the patient satisfied with the effect of physical therapy will not be met when the patient decides to abandon physical therapy or cries that the exercises hurt her. Unmet needs generate feelings. When the therapist is only vaguely aware of his needs and feelings, or completely unaware of them, he tends to form judgments of the patient. The therapist must ask himself:

Have I judged the patient?

Do I regard her as *self-pitying?*

Do I think she is *lazy?*

Do I see her as *trying to get attention?*

Once a person has judged, it is difficult for him to reflect honestly on his own feelings. He focuses on his judgment, not on his feelings. His words then will reflect the judgment and will lead to misunderstanding. In order that the interaction produce genuine understanding, the speaker must resist the temptation to judge, take the time to become aware of needs, and reflect on his own feelings toward the other.

The statement by the therapist, "If you don't try harder and get a better attitude, you will never feel well," does not reveal the therapist's feelings. Potentially, the therapist's remark will not motivate the patient and most assuredly will serve to cast the patient into self-doubt and feelings of resentment toward the therapist. The remark, then, is detrimental to a satisfying relationship between the therapist and the patient and to successful treatment of the patient's symptoms. The therapist must heighten his awareness of the judgments he has made of the patient and of the feelings he experiences toward the patient as a result. By bringing the feelings into awareness, the therapist can take the time to reflect on them before he speaks. He can decide whether he wants to share the feelings or simply be more alert to the feelings and to the way they might influence his behavior toward the patient. Alternatively, he can, with awareness of his feelings, choose to share them with the patient directly. For example,

> I feel concern for you when I see you avoiding the exercises we discussed yesterday.
>
> or
>
> I feel frustrated when it looks like you are not trying very hard.

The health–care provider has to weigh his decision before sharing his feelings directly to the patient. This alternative is possible only when the therapist has taken the time to be aware of his feelings.

Example #2: Doctor and Patient

Frances has not felt well for several months. Her symptoms have increased in severity since her last visit to her doctor. At this appointment Frances is determined to inform the doctor clearly as to her condition. Unfortunately, out of fear that she will be viewed as "one more complaining, neurotic woman," Frances refrains from sharing most of her symptoms and from communicating the intensity of the fatigue she has been feeling.

Doctor: Hello, Frances. How can I help you? What has been happening?
Frances: Well, I haven't been feeling very well, not any bet-

ter than the last time I saw you. It's not too bad, but I think I'm kind of tired.

Doctor: When are you feeling tired? You have to rest more.

Frances: Well, yes, I feel tired then maybe even more than at other times, but I'm tired pretty much all the time.

Doctor: How's your diet? I remember from your last visit you were trying to become more aware that you need a better diet.

Frances: Well, yes, that's true. I have changed somewhat how I eat. Maybe I could even be more careful, I suppose. But, I think that this fatigue is different. You know, different from ordinary feeling tired.

At home, Frances had complained vehemently that she was unreasonably, inexplicably tired. She had cried over the fatigue and seemed determined to describe her symptoms of fatigue so clearly that the doctor would have "to see I'm really suffering." However, at the office Frances fails to communicate the intensity of her lethargy and the doctor is left ignorant of her condition. Frances reflects during a therapy session on her needs, feelings, and judgments during the interaction with her physician.

What are my needs?
To have the doctor see me as different from other complaining women

To be affirmed by the doctor

To be seen as cooperative

What was I feeling?
Vulnerable to his perceptions that I am imagining the fatigue

Timid when faced with his authority

Inadequate to the task of describing my symptoms without doubt

Have I judged the doctor?
Do I regard him as a sexist?

Do I see him as lacking understanding?

Have I judged him as an inflexible authoritarian figure?

Frances recognizes that her feelings of inadequacy and vulnerability have so inhibited her that she has failed to share her symptoms to the degree that she feels them. She has, in fact, minimized them. She has allowed her needs to be liked and affirmed by the doctor to interfere with clear communication of her symptoms. When the feelings and needs that Frances experiences are identified, she is more prepared to communicate clearly with the doctor. For example,

> I need to let you know how bad the fatigue is, but I fear that you will think that I am imagining the fatigue or exaggerating it.

Once the feelings are identified, the patient also has the option of deciding not to share the feelings but also not allowing the fear to inhibit her interaction with the physician. She can, for example, simply say,

> I need to tell you how bad the fatigue has become.

If, after hearing her complaint, the doctor did indeed express suspicion that her fatigue was real, then Frances would need to reflect on her feelings once again. At this point, feeling frustrated and needing to be listened to with trust, Frances might say,

> Doctor, I feel frustrated when you ask about the diet. I was fearful that you would dismiss my fatigue and it seems that you have. I need you to give it your attention so that I can get whatever treatment will help me.

Feelings do not always have to be shared for effective meeting to take place. But the feelings need to be identified or they will control the interaction; in this case, for example, the fear might keep the patient from sharing frustration—it could even lead to another change of doctors when such a change might not be beneficial or necessary.

Example #3: Husband and Wife

June has lupus. She is twenty-nine years old and has been married to Graham for four years. They have discussed having a baby many times, but recently Graham has cut short any conversation on the topic and has appeared irritated whenever June has tried to open up the subject. Determined to "bring the issue to a head," June confronted Graham when they were clearing up after dinner.

June: Graham, what is it with you? You've totally closed me out on talking about getting pregnant. Your job and making money mean more to you than starting a family.

Graham: That's crazy. Plus, you wanted the bigger house, not me.

June: You wanted the house, too. Don't put that all on me.

Graham: Come on. You pushed and pushed for it. Remember the complaining about how small the apartment was?

June: That's not fair. We both wanted out of there.

Graham: Well, we're out, okay. But this place is not going to be paid for by my working nine to five. I'm going upstairs.

June: Great, walk out whenever we need to talk.

These young partners have just had another fruitless argument. Neither really got to his or her feelings, especially feelings about having a baby. They steered away from the potentially explosive issue of pregnancy and argued about the house and money and job. June starts off the exchange with a question loaded with blame:

"What is it with you?"

She follows up with two judgments:

> "You've totally closed me out on talking about getting
> pregnant."
> "Your job and making money mean more to you than
> starting a family."

June's blame and judgment set off feelings within Graham
so that he counterattacks and quickly moves to a safer subject.

> "That's crazy."
> "You wanted the bigger house, not me."

From there on, it is further acting out of feelings with "thrust
and parry."

If June and Graham were to share honestly what they were
really feeling, their interaction might sound something like
this.

June: Graham, I feel confused and hurt when it doesn't seem
like you want to talk about having a baby.

Graham: God knows I want a baby. But I'm afraid that you
are getting very serious about having one. And I'm afraid
of what it might do to you.

June: Well, I get afraid, too. But I want to have a baby more
than I'm afraid of what it might cause.

Graham: I've been too afraid that you would go ahead. I've
been angry at you for being willing to risk your health.
But then I've been angry at the thought of not having
children.

If June and Graham could admit their feelings and share
them with one another, they would see how similar their
feelings and needs are. They would realize their common
fear, their common desire for a child, their need for one
another, and their love. Communicating honestly is a risk,

but it can avoid useless, hurtful acting out of feelings and foster union and understanding.

Steps Toward Direct Sharing of Feelings

Most of us can respond immediately when asked what we are thinking, but we tend to go blank when asked what we are feeling. Though feelings are vitally important to understanding ourselves and others, and though feelings strongly influence our opinions and perceptions as well as our behavior, we are often totally unable to identify them. We have educated vocabularies for expressing our opinions but almost no words to describe what is happening in our emotional lives. We can, however, learn to identify our emotions and to express them without blame or judgment. The following list may be helpful to you as you attempt to identify your feelings and express them.

adventurous	astonished	compassionate
affectionate	aversion	complacent
afraid	awe	composed
agitated	bewildered	concerned
alarm	bitter	confident
alert	blah	confused
alive	blissful	contemptuous
aloof	blue	content
amazed	bored	cool
amused	brave	cooperative
angry	brokenhearted	courageous
anguish	buoyant	credulous
animosity	calm	cross
annoyance	carefree	curious
anxious	cautious	deferential
apathetic	cheerful	defiant
appreciation	choked up	dejected
apprehensive	close	delighted
aroused	cold	dependent
ashamed	comfortable	depressed

despair	exhilarated	hurt
despondent	expansive	immobilized
detached	expectant	impatient
determined	exuberant	inadequate
disappointed	fascinated	independent
discouraged	fearful	indifferent
disgruntled	fidgety	inert
disgusted	firm	infuriated
disheartened	forlorn	inquisitive
dishonest	free	insecure
dislike	friendly	insensitive
dismayed	frightened	inspired
dissatisfied	frisky	intense
distant	frustrated	interested
distressed	furious	intrigued
disturbed	giddy	invigorated
downcast	gloomy	involved
eager	good-humored	irate
ecstatic	grateful	irritated
edgy	gratification	jealous
effervescent	grief	jittery
elated	grief-stricken	joyful
electrified	grumpy	jubilant
embarrassed	guilty	keyed up
embittered	gutless	lonely
encouraged	happy	love
engrossed	hard	loving
enjoyment	hate	mad
enraged	heavy	mean
enthusiastic	helpful	melancholy
envious	helpless	mellow
estranged	hesitant	merry
evasive	horrible	mirthful
exalted	horrified	miserable
exasperated	hostile	mixed up
excited	hot	moved
exhausted	humdrum	open

optimistic	self-assured	tense
overjoyed	sensitive	tepid
overwhelmed	shaky	terrified
panicky	shocked	thankful
paralyzed	silly	thrilled
peaceful	skeptical	timid
pessimistic	soft	tired
pleased	sorrowful	torn
pleasure	sorry	tranquil
powerless	sour	troubled
proud	spellbound	trusting
puzzled	spineless	uncomfortable
radiant	spiritless	unconcerned
rancorous	splendid	uneasy
rapturous	startled	unhappy
relieved	stimulated	upset
reluctant	stretched	uptight
repelled	strong	vacant
resentful	submissive	warm
respectful	sunshiny	weepy
restless	surprised	wide-awake
sad	suspicious	withdrawn
satisfied	sympathetic	woeful
scared	talkative	worried
secure	taut	wretched
seductive	tenderness	

Steps Toward Direct Expression of Feelings

Be sure to state the feelings directly:

I feel *(concerned, frustrated, afraid, hurt, impatient)* (The words "I feel" are followed by an emotion.) As the couple in the following instance demonstrates, such clear expression is not easy. The couple came to see us claiming that the husband's chronic fatigue was destroying their marriage. When they were asked to talk about their feelings regarding this illness, the wife, Myra, began talking to her husband, Bob.

> I think that you are so used to being brave and strong that you can't allow yourself the right to be sad and discouraged over the fatigue.

Myra was sure that she had identified her feelings and had shared them with Bob. Her observation about Bob might be accurate (he did not agree), but her intention had been to share her feelings, not to outline her observations. Instead she had told Bob about Bob. He then angrily disagreed with her. She tried once again to share her feelings.

> You look like you're sad, but when I ask you how you're feeling, you say everything's fine.

Again, her description of their interaction might be accurate, but she focused on Bob; whatever she felt in response to the interaction was absent. She looked frustrated when encouraged to try again to reflect on her *feelings*. This time, however, she paused and, despite her frustration, admitted,

> I guess I'm *afraid* that Bob won't tell me when he's feeling discouraged. I'm *afraid* he'll try to deal with this illness by himself and won't let me in to help him. I think I'm also *scared* that he'll get frustrated and then take it out on me.

As she stated her feelings directly, Myra became more visible. We came to know Myra this time. The first two times she spoke she sounded more like a pseudo-analyst than a woman with strong feelings and needs regarding the man she loved.

Avoid sentences that start with the words "I feel that . . ." or "I feel like. . . ." When the words "I feel" are followed by the word "that" and "like," they usually precede a judgment:

> I feel *that you are lazy*.
> I feel *that you are not trying hard enough*.

I feel *like you don't really care.*
I feel *that the way you are acting is never going to help you.*

Nowhere in these statements are the feelings of the speaker revealed; further, the judgments are stated *as if* they were facts.

At one workshop, we were working with a group of young men and women. Brian, a young man who had expressed much enthusiasm about learning the skills, said, "I want to say what I'm feeling to you, Felicia." Felicia had been fairly quiet throughout the morning workshop and looked at him somewhat warily; however, she appeared open to what he had to say. He leaned forward a bit and said, "I feel that you're shy and a little uptight." The entire group was quiet. We all looked at Brian and back to Felicia. Brian sat up and defensively barked, "What? What did I say? I told her how I felt about her." Brian genuinely believed that he had told Felicia how he felt toward her. When he reflected on his words he noted, "Actually, I had been thinking about Felicia all morning. I have a real problem with people who are quiet. I kind of assume that they're snobs. But I was trying not to judge Felicia as a snob so I figured maybe she's shy." Brian was lost in his thoughts when he spoke to Felicia, and, indeed, he expressed his thoughts, not his feelings. If your intention is to express an emotion, beware of the words, "I feel that . . ." or "I think that . . ." or "I feel like. . . ." Inevitably, they will lead you away from your feelings.

Avoid sharing *your* feelings by using the words "we," "all of us," "everyone":

> *We all* feel frustrated with your lack of progress.
> *Everyone* thinks that you are not trying.
> *All of us* wish that you would get a better attitude.

Resist the temptation to depersonalize *your* feelings by speaking for others. It is worthwhile for you to reflect on your need to say "we" rather than "I." Ask yourself, "What am I feeling?" For example, are you afraid that the person listening to you will become angry and so you attempt to support your feelings by indicating that others feel the same way? Sharing *your* feelings by commencing the statement with "we" is not fair to the listener, who is trying to listen to *your* feelings and then must deal with the implication that "everyone" feels the same way. It is quite an assumption to believe that more than one person feels exactly the same emotion.

Be sure to keep the focus on yourself when you are sharing your feelings. When you shift the focus from yourself by using pronouns other than "I" or adding the word "that" and a judgment, you have placed the focus on the other. Be aware of your intentions. Do you really want to share your feelings or do you want to blame, accuse, or judge? During a recent communications workshop that we were conducting for business men and women, one fellow who had grown increasingly frustrated during the session blurted, "You know, when you're trying to talk to someone, you don't want to have to analyze all your thoughts. You have to be spontaneous." We could be fairly sure that he was referring to himself, but he chose the global "you" instead of the personal "I" when he spoke. He admitted later that he was angry when he thought that the skills we were teaching would restrict him rather than free him to speak openly. He was concerned, though, that he would appear disrespectful, so he spoke in what he felt were "safer" intellectual terms.

Be sure to be aware of your perceptions and interpretations of observed behavior.

A perception is composed of two parts: a sense observation of something or someone; and an interpretation of what has been observed. For example:

1. I observe you speaking more slowly and carefully than usual.

2. I interpret your behavior to mean that you are nervous.

My observation may not be accurate and my interpretation may be way off the mark. Yet, I do have this perception of the way that you are speaking. That perception triggers feelings in me, for instance, compassion or concern.

Another example:

1. I see that you are wearing a black dress.
2. I interpret your behavior to mean that you are in mourning.

Again, my perception evokes feelings. In this case I might feel protective feelings toward you or I might feel disappointment if I had hoped that we were going dancing. Remember, it is not a fact that you are in mourning. It is simply my perception and interpretation. Indeed, you might just believe that you look good in black. It might not even be a fact that you are dressed in black. Color-blind people all tell stories of mistaken observations regarding color. What we see, hear, sense, and interpret is our perception—it is not necessarily reality or fact.

You need to keep in mind the fallibility of your perceptions when you share the feelings that these perceptions generate. Using words such as "seems," "looks like," or "appears" guides you in the direction of sharing perceptions rather than judgments of fact.

> "I felt caring for you while you were speaking. You *seemed* to be nervous."
> "I felt compassion for you when I saw you wearing black. You *appeared* to be in mourning.
> "I feel worried when you *seem* to stop trying."
> "I feel concern for you when you *look* to be unhappy."

Avoid language that makes your observation sound like fact. Remember that your observations are only your perceptions. You have a right to these perceptions. You have a right to the feelings that accompany these perceptions. But your perceptions are not statements of what is reality—just what it seems like to you. Someone else may view what you perceive in an entirely different fashion. The following statements are judgments:

> I feel worried when *you don't try hard*.
> I feel irritated because *you are ignoring my suggestion*.
> I feel concern for you because *you are so unhappy*.

We can be convinced that we know exactly what someone is feeling, but it is safer to assume that we do not know someone's feelings before they are expressed. In a counseling session, Marguerite said to her mother, "I am mad because I can tell you're really irritated with me and it's pretty obvious that you're angry." It is easy to imagine that an argument would ensue from such a statement. In this example, Marguerite did share her feelings, but her perceptions of her mother would have been received more readily if she had prefaced them with "It *seems* like you are angry," or "You *look* to me like you are angry." For Marguerite, as for all of us, speaking in this manner takes discipline, particularly when we are convinced that we truly do know how someone feels. When we cautioned Marguerite to avoid stating her perceptions as if they were facts, she responded, "I know my mother. Believe me, I know when she's mad at me." Her mother said quietly, "No, not really, Marguerite. Sometimes I'm confused or I'm anxious. At other times I'm scared. You seem to take all of my feelings as anger."

Be sure to identify the person's behavior with a specific time when you are offering your feelings. Feelings are "time specific":

> I felt (happy, angry, hurt) *when* (you came into the room).

Notice, for example, Carolyn's statement "I feel frustrated when I describe my symptoms and you tell me I just need to rest more." She identifies specifically *when* she feels frustrated. This is what we mean when we say feelings are "time specific." They change from moment to moment, from person to person, and from situation to situation. Carolyn may feel frustrated in this instance, but with another person, at another time, and with a different perception, she will feel other emotions. Identifying the feeling with specificity as to time and perceived behavior avoids judgment.

Conclusion

Making the effort to communicate in the manner we have outlined can result in enormous benefits for the individual and for his relationships. Rigorous focusing on our feelings and needs is a pathway to self-knowledge, since feelings are revelatory of needs, values, and beliefs. When we recognize fear, rejection, or delight and admit the reason for the feeling, we come to know ourselves. Denial of such feelings leads to self-deception and to lack of integrity. We might not like to feel afraid before making a presentation or giving a report in front of a group, but the feeling tells us about our needs in that situation—needs for respect, approval, or job security. It tells us of our perceptions of the group, for example, as friendly, powerful, or hostile, as well as of our own sense of ourselves in the group, for example, as insecure, respected, or feared.

One of our clients, Rick, was out of work for three months with a severe attack of chronic fatigue. He described his thoughts and feelings about returning to work.

> At first, I really thought of not returning to my company. I pictured some other job that would not demand so much, maybe a job working at home. I kept thinking that I owed it to the company to be totally on the job, giving 150 percent, or not to return at all. I owe the company a lot. It's been good to me. But, then I did what you've been telling me—I tried to get to my feelings and figure out what I was really feeling and why.

I've never felt as smart as a lot of the other guys. I get the job done by staying at it till it's finished even if I'm up all night. I felt afraid that I couldn't do that anymore and I'd let the company down, especially my boss. I couldn't stand that. I've had to look at this feeling of gratitude to the company and to my boss and how it's encouraged me to be loyal to the point of hurting myself and my family. Plus, I've had to look at my feelings of inferiority and what they do to me. It's not going to be easy, but I've got to go back to work with a different attitude.

Awareness of our feelings also liberates us from conditioned reactions that are often self-defeating as well as destructive to relationships. We might not be able to control an immediate feeling of fear when offered a new challenge, but we can control our behaviors, such as immediate withdrawal or rejection of opportunity. We might feel intimidated by someone, but if we are aware of the feeling we can choose not to play the little-girl role, or the bad-boy role, or the braggart role that we adopt when afflicted with feelings of fear and inferiority. Separating the feeling from the behavior leads to greater self-control and greater freedom.

Another freedom fostered by self-awareness is the freedom gained by focusing on self-improvement rather than on the improvement of others. If we feel impatient when a friend is ten minutes late for a meeting, we can admit the feeling to ourselves and then resolve the feeling either by reflecting that we tend to be compulsive about time or by remembering that our friend is seldom late. Or we can share the feeling, admitting that it is difficult for us to wait, even admitting that we are hurt if we read the lateness as not caring about us. We don't have to react to the situation by lecturing or blaming or conveying annoyance. We can focus on ourselves and be real instead of focusing on the friend and being obnoxious.

Relationships are made strong by self-revelation and empathy, behaviors that nurture trust. To reveal our innermost feelings, needs, beliefs, and reflections involves risk of rejection. We might be misunderstood, laughed at, judged as weak, sick, or sad. We reveal ourselves at risk to ourselves. But when we take the risk, most of the time we experience the satisfaction of being honest. We trust ourselves more and know that we can be trusted. Very often our sharing evokes self-sharing by the other. Role-playing tends to prompt role-playing; honesty tends to invite honesty. Honest self-revelation does not mean talking *about* self: our history, what we did on vacation, what diet we are on. Such sharing usually involves little risk and is easily managed to elicit the responses we desire—awe, envy, respect. Self-revelation risks sharing our immediate feelings, needs, reflections. It demands self-knowledge and self-awareness while it promotes their growth. When we admit and share our feelings, we come to know ourselves; when we are heard and understood, we come to accept ourselves.

One woman who knows she has tested HIV positive described her experience of coming to know herself by becoming more conscious of her feelings.

> All I knew for a long time was that I felt miserable. I stormed around the house one day or stayed in bed till noon on another day. I would fantasize about how I was going to radically change my life. I dreamed of running away to a country area and living in a little house all by myself. I would have very few possessions and everything would be simple. Then I would feel hopeless because I knew that I wasn't going to run away and I knew that I couldn't get away from the specter of knowing that I was diagnosed HIV positive.
>
> When you challenged me to go deeper beyond the fantasies and temptations to run away, at first I was pissed off. How would you like to have the threat of AIDS in your life? The last thing I wanted to know was how I really felt. But you were so persistent and finally, *finally* I know now what I'm feeling. I am so angry. Angry at this disease. Angry at my ex-boyfriend. Angry at soci-

ety for regarding me as a pariah. And I'm so scared, so scared of being alone. Isn't that ironic, considering that I wanted to run away and live by myself?

This may sound strange to people who are terrified about AIDS, but I feel more peaceful now. My restlessness is gone. I'm still angry and lonely but I can live with myself. I have to remind myself every day to stay with my feelings and not to go into the fantasies but in some way I think I know myself more now and I have more control.

18

Hearing What Is Said

When I say that I enjoy hearing someone, I mean, of course, hearing deeply. I mean that I hear the words, the thoughts, the feeling tones, the personal meaning, even the meaning that is below the conscious intent of the speaker. Sometimes, too, in a message which superficially is not very important, I hear a deep human cry that lies buried and unknown far below the surface of the person.

Carl R. Rogers

Listening may seem as easy and as natural a behavior as breathing. Indeed, hearing is natural. But truly listening to another person's feelings is something entirely different, something far more difficult than simply being sure that the ears are free of obstructions. When anyone expresses himself, the intention, or hope, is that someone will listen. Someone hearing him intends to listen. One talks, the other listens. Sounds easy. So what interferes? Why is it that so many teen-agers say that their parents do not listen, and why is it that so many parents do not experience their children listening to them? One of the most predictable complaints of a failed marriage is, "He/she never listened to me." Evidently, despite a sometimes desperate need for listening, it does not occur.

We are referring to empathic listening, listening that truly communicates understanding. Such listening requires more than simply hearing the words of another person. It demands that you place your own feelings on hold and resist urges to advise, dismiss, defend, or explain away the other's feelings. It means putting yourself in the service of the other, with a determination to respect the person's feelings without judging those feelings or the person having them.

For many reasons we need to talk about what goes on inside us, to admit our feelings to ourselves, and to share them with someone who will listen. The individual trying to cope with invisible chronic illness feels this need with an urgency hard to exaggerate. The central feeling generated by ICI is fear: fear of being ill, of abandonment, of being insane, of the future, of disfigurement, of death. There are myriad other feelings: anger, rage, discouragement, despair, loneliness, sadness, guilt, shame. The person suffocating with these feelings needs to talk and be understood as much as she needs air. She has to learn to listen to herself and to those she loves. She also needs those close to her to learn how to listen.

Listening with understanding is an act of love. But it is also a skill that can be learned. In order to learn the skill, you need to identify your nonlistening behaviors, that is, all the ways that you respond that do not convey understanding. Then you need to acquire the skill of listening and to practice, practice, practice. In this chapter, we will outline behaviors essential to listening, behaviors that convey empathy. We will also suggest nonlistening behaviors to avoid. Good intentions are necessary to become a good listener, but those intentions need to be applied to the challenging task of changing old habits and practicing new behaviors.

One patient told us, "I was determined to listen to my husband, to really try to understand him. So we got together one night and he talked and talked about his fatigue. I didn't say a word. I just kept my mouth shut—no advice, nothing. But, you know, he still wasn't satisfied." This woman was on the right track. She had learned that her proclivity for giving advice and talking too much contributed to her husband's reticence to talk. Her husband needed her to be quiet so that he could talk, but he also needed something that assured him that she had taken in all that he had shared.

Listening involves attending to the other person and allowing that person to talk, but it also requires letting the person know exactly what has been heard. This is when listening becomes "active."

The listener has to respond in his own words, telling the person who has shared, "This is what I heard." Then, once the listener responds, the person who shared originally has the opportunity to clarify. The process demands discipline, commitment, and skill.

Example 1: Friend and Patient

Tom talked to us about a conversation that left him feeling very dissatisfied. He was surprised by this, since he had looked forward to talking with his friend and had always felt comfortable with him. He had not shared the fact that his daughter was diagnosed with CMT with anyone else, so he felt discouraged that when he shared it with this friend, he felt more embarrassed than relieved. He narrated their conversation to us.

Tom: I didn't find out that I had CMT until I was in my late twenties. Now the doctor tells us that Sarah, who is only eight years old, has CMT. I wanted to die when I heard it. I can't bear the thought that I gave her something that will make her life difficult.

Friend: Are you sure she has it?

Tom: The doctor says that she definitely does. She doesn't exhibit many symptoms but we knew something was wrong.

Friend: She'll be all right. Look at you. Your life isn't limited much.

Tom: Yeah, that's true. But what's killing me is that, however she's affected, it's my fault.

Friend: God, Tom, you didn't do it on purpose. You want everything for her. I want everything for my kids, too. I feel bad when I think I have failed them in some way.

Tom: I know, I know. But I can't get over this guilt I feel.
Friend: She'll be fine, Tom. You've got to stop thinking about it.
Tom: Yes, I know, but I can't. I can't look at her without being flooded with guilt.

Tom's friend seemed well-intentioned. He obviously wanted to comfort Tom. Unfortunately, his desire to comfort interfered with his ability to listen. Notice that to the very end of their conversation, Tom was still talking about his feelings. If his friend's intention was to comfort, he doesn't seem to have succeeded. If his intention was to listen to Tom, he failed. There are a number of things that Tom's friend did other than listen.

He asked a question: "Are you sure she has it?"

There is nothing inherently wrong with asking a question. Questions are necessary to obtain information or to satisfy our curiosity. Inquisitiveness can show apparent interest, which is sometimes genuine. However, when our intention is to listen to another person, more often than not questions are distracting. Tom's friend was satisfying his own need to move away from the uncomfortable subject of Tom's feelings of guilt. If he was truly doubtful about the diagnosis, he could ask later. His job as listener was to attend first to Tom's feelings.

He attempted to offer comfort: "She'll be all right." "She'll be fine."

Tom's friend seems to want Tom to feel better. But if he stopped to examine what he has said, he might be struck by the remarkable assumptions in his statements. Surely, he does not think that he can predict the future. Probably, like many of us, he offers facile words of comfort when faced with another person's pain. Apparently he is hearing Tom's distress, but he does not acknowledge it. Instead of letting

Tom know clearly that he has heard his feelings, he tries to comfort. Even when phrases such as "Don't worry, everything will be fine," or "Things will get better," are well-intentioned, they tend to be more irritating than comforting to someone who wants to be heard. We have to learn to trust that one of the greatest sources of comfort is listening.

He gave advice: "You've got to stop thinking about it."

This may, in fact, be good advice. Constant rumination over a worrisome thought leads only to anxiety. But when someone needs to be heard, advice is a cheap substitute for listening. Advice frequently puts a person on the defensive and prompts him to respond with, "Yes, but . . ."

"You have to stop thinking about it."
    "Yes, but I can't."
    "Yes, but I tried that."
    "Yes, but that won't help me solve . . ."
    "Yes, but I thought of that."

We like to give advice more than receive it. In many instances giving advice reflects the listener's discomfort with what he is hearing. We have to learn to trust not only that listening is a comfort but also that by listening we help the other person come to his own solution.

He shifted the focus to himself: "I want everything for my kids, too. I feel bad when I think I have failed them."

When someone shares with us, it tends to trigger reminders of our own situation. Those reminders can lead to empathy, but too often they can sidetrack the listener to his own story before he has taken the time to listen fully to the speaker. Tom's friend shifted too quickly to talk about himself. Perhaps he was trying to encourage or comfort Tom, but Tom did not feel encouraged or comforted. He felt frustrated. He needed more time to talk before he could listen to his friend.

At some point the focus of the conversation does have to shift to the listener; otherwise relationships would be one-sided. But it is best to be guided by the maxim, "Listen first."

One listening tactic is to repeat back in your own words what you have heard the speaker say. Keeping this behavior in mind can free you from a thousand other nonlistening behaviors. When someone has spoken and you start to respond, *hold it,* and make sure that you are offering back in your own words what you have just heard. This behavior might seem unnatural or awkward. With practice it can become quite natural. No skill is learned without passing through a time of clumsiness or awkwardness. Remember, hold your immediate reaction when responding to what someone has said, and offer back what you have just heard. Use a formula for a while to assist you; for example, "What I heard you say was . . ." or "It sounds like you said . . ." or "I think I heard you say. . . ." Your attention is on the speaker, not on your reaction.

Relating back to the speaker what you have heard does not mean that you are agreeing with him. Agreement is not the issue at the moment of listening. What you are doing is turning your eyes, your ears, your attention onto the speaker and his words. At this moment you are not judging him or his message; you are not agreeing or disagreeing, approving or disapproving. You are simply making sure that what you have heard is what he meant to say. It helps to use words such as "It sounds like" when you are demonstrating listening. These words imply that what you are about to say is what you *think* you have heard rather than exactly what the speaker said. Listening requires humility. Your voice must contain a certain tentativeness that communicates to the sharer that he is the ultimate judge of his feelings.

Steps Toward Effective Empathic Listening

Learning to listen is not easy. We have all developed habits of behavior, habits of reacting when another speaks that, like many habits, are "bad habits." These habitual behaviors have to be identified and seen to be ineffective ways of really connecting with another person. We would all like to be respected as good listeners, but few of us are. Yet listening is a skill like playing the piano or hitting a tennis ball. The skill of listening can be learned. Once we have identified what we do instead of listening (give advice, ask questions that serve our own needs more than the speaker's, talk about ourselves, respond with "me too" identification, focus on what we are going to say when the speaker stops, and so on), then we are ready to listen. The following specific steps, when taken with good will and the desire to really understand the speaker, can lead to genuine meeting.

Be sure to focus your attention on the *feelings* that the person is expressing. This is where you need to start if your intention is to truly hear. You want to communicate to the person what you have heard, and you do this by focusing first on the feelings that you believe you have heard.

> It sounds like you feel *(impatient, afraid, guilty, disappointed)*.

In the example of Tom and his friend, after listening to Tom's statement about his own illness and his reaction to hearing of his daughter's illness, the friend might have responded:

> You sound like you feel sad and guilty at the thought of being responsible for your daughter's illness.

Responding in this way, the friend reveals that he is really trying to hear what Tom is experiencing. He is not trying to talk him out of anything or give advice or talk about himself. He is with Tom and ready to hear what Tom is feeling.

Avoid asking questions. Listen to what the speaker is saying and what the speaker is feeling. The listener can be distracted easily by seeking details regarding the issue at hand.

It is important to listen first to the feelings and later clarify details. Asking a question tends to introduce the listener's interests and agenda and to shift the speaker from his original focus. Only after the person has truly been understood and indicates some satisfaction at being heard are questions appropriate.

In the example above, the friend's question, "Are you sure she has it?" leads Tom away from what *he* seems to be trying to share about *his* pain in hearing about his daughter's illness to a focus on the reliability of diagnosis. The friend's question is an opening salvo in an effort to make Tom feel better. In order to listen, the friend has to drop his well-meaning agenda and focus on listening.

Be sure to allow the speaker the opportunity to clarify his feelings. If you have made an effort to hear the person, then pause to see whether the person appears to be satisfied. Often, if a person feels heard, his behavior will demonstrate his satisfaction. He will nod his head or say, "That's just what I meant," or smile. But if he does not experience being understood, he will need to clarify. If you have shown the person that you are trying to hear accurately even though you are not positive that you know exactly what he is trying to say, the speaker will continue the conversation by saying something such as, "That's not exactly what I was feeling," or "You heard part of it but there is more." Again, to listen in this fashion requires humility. You can't have a vested interest in being affirmed for listening accurately.

Avoid offering comfort too quickly. When a person shares feelings that reveal suffering, it is natural to want to offer comfort. Indeed, the person may need comfort, but once again, listen first. Be sure that you have taken the time to listen as closely as possible to the speaker's feelings.

The listener must be aware of his own feelings, which may cause a "knee-jerk" comforting remark, as, for example, when the friend says, "She'll be all right. Look at you. Your life isn't limited so much." Tom's friend needs to listen to his own feelings as he listens to Tom. Is he feeling *uncomfortable* at hearing Tom's guilt? Does he feel *impatient* with Tom for not letting go of the guilt? Does he feel *anxiety* as Tom opens up? The listener's vigilant awareness of his own feelings requires a discipline that comes with practice.

Avoid telling your own story. Remember, when listening, keep the focus on the speaker. Whatever the person has shared may immediately trigger the listener's own memories of a similar situation—the reflexive "me too" reaction. For example, if Tom were sharing his feelings of guilt to a father who also feels guilt over his children's diagnosis of CMT, Tom may well remind him of his own feelings of guilt. If the listener shifts too quickly into a "me too" version of Tom's feelings, he will leave Tom to talk about himself.

Had Tom's friend been focused on listening instead of reassuring, their interaction might have gone something like this,

Tom: I didn't find out that I had CMT until I was in my late twenties. Now the doctor tells us that Sarah, who is only eight years old, has CMT. I wanted to die when I heard it. I can't bear the thought that I gave her something that will make her life difficult.

Friend: It sounds like you feel horrible at the thought of Sarah suffering and guilty at knowing she probably inherited the illness from you.

Tom: Exactly, it's awful. I didn't have to put up with CMT until I was an adult. She's only eight. And then, I think I am responsible.

Friend: *(Still listening and checking his desire to tell Tom that it's not his fault)* It seems like you dread the thought of what she might have to suffer and that you feel terrible guilt that instead of being able to give her all that's good in life, you may have given her your illness.

Tom: That's it. God, I don't want her to suffer in any way. She's so innocent. So adorable.

Friend: Tom, I hear how much you love her and how painful it is to think she'll suffer due to your illness.

Tom: (*Silent for a while*) I do feel guilty, even though it's not really my fault. It's just you want your kids to have everything and not to suffer.

Friend: I appreciate your sharing with me what means so much to you. I don't have the same thing happening with me and my children. But I can identify with your love, and I know I share that sense of wanting to keep harm away from them and knowing I won't always be able to do that. Anyway, Tom, I think you're a great father.

By listening, the friend has come to know Tom better, has met him where he is at the moment, has allowed Tom to "get it all out," and has become closer to his friend and to himself. Listening promotes meeting.

Example 2: Sister and Patient

Katy, who has lupus, came with her sister for a counseling session. Katy's sister wanted to understand how her sister was dealing with the disease. Just before the session began, they were chatting about their plans for the day. By the time the session began Katy's sister had tears in her eyes and Katy had turned her chair away from her sister and was staring out the window. This was their brief interaction.

Katy: What do you want to do after we finish here?

Sister: I'd like to go shopping first and then have lunch. After that we could go to the new beach area that has just been opened.

Katy: I don't know. It sounds like fun, but I don't think I can do all that.

Sister: Why? You look fine. I thought you were feeling well. Don't you feel well?

Katy: I don't think I ever feel well. I just meant that I'm feeling better than I did before.

Sister: Maybe you really don't want to spend the whole day with me.

Katy: No, I do want to be with you. I just get tired very easily. And you have to remember the sun is dangerous for me.

Sister: I remember. Do you think I haven't been paying attention? I just thought that since it's a cool day, you could go to the beach.

Katy and her sister failed to interact in a way that left them feeling satisfied or enthusiastic about their plans for their day. Katy's sister did not listen to Katy effectively. What did she do other than listen?

> She is defensive: "Maybe you really don't want to spend the whole day with me." "I remember. Do you think I haven't been paying attention?"

Katy's sister intended to be as considerate of Katy as possible, to the point of joining Katy in this therapy session to learn how she could help her. As a consequence of wanting so deeply to be a positive force in Katy's life, she was vulnerable to any remark that suggested she was not. She heard Katy's words as critical of her, felt vulnerable, and responded defensively.

When we think that we hear an attack, criticism, or rejection in someone's words, we respond defensively. It makes sense to prepare to defend when we think that we are being attacked. The key, of course, is, "When we *think* that we hear an attack." Just as Katy's sister has to learn to listen, we have to learn to listen and "check out" what we think we have heard from the speaker. More often than not, if we discipline ourselves to listen and actively demonstrate that we heard accurately, we will hear the person's feelings rather than an attack.

Katy and her sister made a second attempt to discuss their

plans. This time Katy shared her feelings more directly and her sister listened instead of defending herself.

Katy: I would like to do something after we finish here, but I'm afraid I won't have the energy and I'm afraid you'll be disappointed if we don't go to the beach.

Sister: It sounds like you really would enjoy doing something with me after we leave, but you're anxious that you'll get tired and then I won't want to be with you.

Katy: Well, yes, I am anxious about getting tired, but I'm not worried that you won't want to be with me. I am worried that you'll be disappointed.

Sister: Oh, I think I understand. You seem worried that I won't enjoy myself it we can't do much or go to the beach and then I'll be disappointed.

Katy: Yes, that's it exactly.

Asking questions, being defensive, focusing on self, advising, and offering superficial comfort are not forms of listening. Very often they instead reveal, in an indirect manner, the listener's feelings. A listener who is uncomfortable hearing a friend's guilt may try to alleviate that guilt by providing advice. A listener who fears he is being accused of something will be defensive. And a listener who is not trying to hear the feelings of the other will focus on details and ask questions. It is a disquieting, sometimes terribly discouraging experience to share with someone who is not listening. The listener who wants to provide the rich, satisfying experience of being heard must be aware of his own feelings, place them on hold, and focus on the feelings of the person talking.

Example 3: Family and Patient

Ann, who described her interaction with her physical therapist in Chapter 17, returned home to her family. Her husband, Kevin, and their sons, Dennis and Daniel, were at home when she arrived. From Ann's tearful narration, we were able to piece together the following interaction.

Kevin: Hi, Ann. How was the physical therapy?

Ann: Awful. I'm not sure if I should go anymore. It's costing so much money; I feel worse than I did before and today he had the nerve to say that I should try harder and get a better attitude.

Kevin: Maybe he's right.

Ann: What do you mean by that?

Kevin: It wouldn't hurt if you would approach this with a positive attitude.

Ann: You never take my side. You are so ready to assume that I won't try hard.

Dennis: Lay off her, Dad. She's had a bad day.

Daniel: You're a fine one to talk, Dennis. You were happy to make her drive you to school this morning.

Dennis: You're not such a saint yourself.

Kevin: Would you guys leave the room. You're not helping your mother by arguing.

Daniel: I think we should have the right to talk about this.

Ann: None of you are helping me. You don't understand what I'm going through.

Such family interactions, fraught with misunderstandings, occur all too frequently. Everyone leaves the room disgruntled and discouraged. Dennis and Daniel may well want to help their mother, but their feelings of helplessness and guilt interfere with listening to her. They do not share their feelings and what they do say starts an argument. Kevin may be frustrated with what seems to him Ann's lack of a positive attitude toward physical therapy. And Ann may be discouraged at not feeling any improvement in her condition. Yet she does not share her discouragement and it is not heard.

If the family members were more aware of their feelings and more skilled in listening, their interaction might have sounded like this,

Kevin: Hi, Ann. How was the physical therapy?

Ann: I don't know. I feel very discouraged. I'm not feeling better and I'm aware of how much it is costing. Plus, he told me I should try harder and get a better attitude.

Kevin: (*Aware of his feeling of frustration that Ann seems negative, holds his feeling and tries to understand.*) It sounds like you feel really disheartened and frustrated that you're not feeling improvement and then you must feel either hurt or angry at the therapist?

Ann: Kevin, it's so hard. I've gone week after week. I've done the exercises. It's like I've gone nowhere. I don't want to be negative, but I feel almost helpless.

Kevin: I know it's got to feel very discouraging to put so much effort out and feel no result. Then his comment must have hurt.

Dennis: I feel bad, Mom. I wish you felt better.

Daniel: Me too. I'll work out with you—you know, do your exercises with you. Maybe that would help.

Here the focus has stayed on Ann's feelings of discouragement and hurt. Her husband has listened rather than scolded or judged. The boys have demonstrated their love and care. As a family they are united in response to one's pain instead of divided in a way that exacerbates Ann's pain while making all of them suffer.

Conclusion

When we really listen we experience the same liberating effect as the one being heard. Listening frees us from quick presumptions and knee-jerk reactions. When a friend says, "I feel terrible. The pain is right back in my neck and head. I can't live like this," our first reaction is to try to encourage or motivate or even to criticize a "negative attitude." But when we "hold it" and listen, we can hear discouragement or fear and connect with our friend in a true and comforting way. We are freed from reacting, and our friend is freed not only from having to hear this reaction but also from isola-

tion. He is encouraged to trust our response. Listening provides for the one speaking a safe space to share himself, to
come to understand himself, to be himself.

When we attempt to say something that we really mean—
a belief, an opinion, a reflection, a feeling—we seldom find
the right words immediately. We need the opportunity to
speak freely, not distracted by the other's thought or defensive about his reaction. We need room to clarify and to
reformulate our thoughts or feelings. When we experience
understanding, we are freed to share more clearly, to get
deeper into ourselves. Listening is a key that frees us to share
ourselves, and in so doing, we come to understand ourselves. In The Transparent Self, Sidney Jourard describes the
effect of putting ourselves into words and then putting ourselves in these words out toward another: ". . . no man can
come to know himself except as an outcome of disclosing
himself to another person."[1] In becoming "transparent" to
the other, we become "transparent" to ourselves and thus
come to see ourselves more clearly. The empathy of the
listener, then, gives to us the opportunity to know ourselves.

When we experience someone listening to us without
judging or prodding, we develop trust in the other, trust
that frees us to share more of ourselves. Frequently, the one
with whom we yearn to share ourselves and by whom we
need to be understood is busy doing something else—advising or blaming, talking about himself or something else. So
we stop trying to share. The result is often a desperate loneliness.

Julie, who suffers from post-polio syndrome, told us in
tears of the distance she experiences from her husband.

> I used to try to tell him about what goes on inside of
> me, but I'd sense him tensing up. He didn't want to
> listen. He'd start to lecture me if he thought I was com-
> plaining. If he thought I was criticizing my doctor or
> someone who had been insensitive, he'd defend them.
> I've started talking much more to my mother or my

best friend. But I'm not sure that's good either. I don't know where we're going in our marriage.

Julie's husband, Don, told us in a joint session with her that he was afraid to respond to her since she would immediately start arguing with him. He had not realized that his responses were not empathic ones. He meant well and tried to help. Yet he viewed her as very negative. He needed to learn that his fears, and even impatience, were causing him to react rather than to listen. Then Julie reacted to his reaction— consequently both were hurt and frustrated. Both needed to listen. Julie needed to hear his efforts, even his fear and impatience. Don needed to stop advising and defending and learn to listen.

Relating honestly, being totally present to the being of the other, is for us a behavioral description of loving. Speaking the truth of our feelings, needs, and perceptions and listening for these in the other are the essence of being present to ourselves and to the other. Such presence is liberating. One of our clients paid us the highest tribute when she wrote:

> I was quite anxious about going to my first workshop and meeting you. As it turned out, I was terrified by the experience and of its goal of closeness, but I wasn't afraid of you. You were so solid, so consistent and so real that it was as if some part of me that was real too came out of nowhere and I responded to you. In the years since that has never changed. I think that is one of your gifts, it's like you can spot whatever is true and sound within a person and then that's what you talk to, focus on, and nurture. When I am with you or in your company, I think I become the person I was always supposed to have been. It's easy to be real.

We challenge ourselves to live up to such trust. We challenge our clients and you, our readers, to speak your truth consistently and courageously and to listen deeply and selflessly. We *can* be more whole and more free and more freeing.

19

Managing Stress Associated with ICI

Slow down, you move too fast
You got to make the morning last.

Simon and Garfunkel

Doctor to patient: The tests don't show anything. Your problem seems to be stress. Maybe it would be a good idea to see a psychiatrist and talk things out.

Doctor to patient: These symptoms are all signs of stress. I want you to take these twice a day and let's see how you do. Try to get a lot of rest and see if you can't get away to that place you have in New Hampshire.

"Stress" is all too often the catch-all diagnosis delivered by doctors who cannot explain the symptoms their patients describe. For the patient yearning for a clear-cut diagnosis and treatment, the "stress explanation" is a discouraging dismissal. It is a diagnosis impossible to refute and infuriating to receive. The message implied or inferred is: *There's nothing really wrong with you that good mental health and exercise wouldn't cure.*

The stress message proffered by doctors, family members, and friends as helpful advice usually provokes just what it cautions against—stress. There might be wisdom in the suggestions to relax, be sensible, and exercise, but for the person wrestling with self-doubt, pain, and fatigue, the advice can be very irritating.

In this concluding chapter we explore stress not as the

explanation for invisible chronic illness but as a reaction to perceived threat within the bodies of ICI sufferers. For the ICI patient the perceived threats are those that threaten her well-being; this well-being is most at risk when certain basic needs are unfulfilled. Here we focus upon those needs and summarize ways and means of meeting them.

Acute and Chronic Stress

During a workshop, Mary made a presentation to a group of officers at an oil company. She had administered the Myers–Briggs Type Inventory (a personality inventory) to them and now had three hours to lead them to further understanding of themselves and of one another by means of the test results. On the day preceding the presentation, Mary felt nervous. Would she make the presentation clear and entertaining? Would the officers be interested and involved? Would they respond warmly to her and openly to one another? The morning of her talk, Mary did not feel hungry for breakfast, her mouth felt dry, and she was rather restless. As soon as Mary began to talk to the officers, her nervousness vanished, her adrenalin pumped energy into her words and expression; she was animated, informative, alert. The officers responded to her energy and very quickly the group was alive with questions, insights, and laughter. The group seemed surprised at how rapidly the three hours passed.

Mary had experienced acute stress; that is, stress specific to a perceived threat to well-being. Acute stress is generally brief and resolved if the specific threat is confronted successfully. Such stresses make life interesting. They occur whenever we attempt something that connects to a need to achieve and to be successful: hosting a dinner party, making a presentation, playing a tennis match. Similarly, our bodies register stress through rapid heartbeat, flushed cheeks, or cheeks drained of color when we have to react quickly to a perceived danger: a car swerving into our lane or a baby about to fall out of a chair. The threat is specific and definable, and the stress we feel passes once the incident is resolved.

Our bodies have reacted "on alert" to the perceived danger: rush of adrenalin, quickened pulse, dilated pupils. With the passing of the danger, our bodies revert to their relaxed state.

Chronic stress refers to the debilitating condition of "on alert" minds and bodies that do not revert to an easy, relaxed mode. Battle fatigue and burnout are results of chronic stress—for too long a period, the organism has not been able to function in a calm, smooth, satisfying way. The result can be serious malfunctioning of mind and body. Hypertension, irritability, nervous tics, and depression are some of the signs of chronic stress.

Chronic stress results when one or more major need is not met over a sustained period. The following are needs that are typically threatened as a result of ICI:

> to be healthy
> to feel well
> to achieve
> to be understood
> to be supported
> to be loved
> to love
> to know and accept self; to be authentic

As we discussed in the previous chapters, the person suffering with invisible chronic illness seldom feels well and his ability to achieve is constantly threatened. Often he suffers from not experiencing understanding and support and fears that his love is not valued or needed, while fearing that he himself is hardly lovable. For the ICI patient such deprivation often triggers pervasive chronic stress.

Managing Stress

In the face of persistent threat to her well-being, the person with ICI can reduce stress by learning to take good care of herself, that is, to nourish herself by knowing her needs and meeting them. Some of these needs are discussed below.

THE NEED TO FEEL WELL

An advertisement for Geritol used to proclaim that if you have your health, you have just about everything. Well, with ICI, you don't have your health. Your daily stress involves not feeling well, and because of the incurable nature of ICI, you can't look forward to the threat passing. But you can learn to live with poor health and do all in your power—mind and body—to feel as well as possible. Certain proven methods for reducing stress directly address physical symptoms. Involving yourself in such activities also affects the mental and emotional dimension of feeling well. A further important benefit is the sense of reducing helplessness. Positive action tends to feed a positive attitude. Involvement in activities ranging from yoga to meditation to cultural events can all become part of managing the stress surrounding the complex experience of chronic intermittent bouts of pain and fatigue. We will discuss six of the ways that you might lessen the stress you experience while promoting a sense of well-being.

Exercise and Play   All work and no play can make Jack not only a dull boy but also a sick one. More and more researchers and theorists point to the need for exercise to promote health. Even a small amount of exercise can increase energy and reduce hypertension. Many clients have told us how much better they feel after going for a run or walk or doing low-impact aerobics. Some, like vascular surgeon Irv Dardik,[1] believe that very vigorous exercise that raises the heart rate and is followed by immediate rest or recovery is deeply healing for persons suffering with chronic illness.

When you are ill, however, it is natural to stop exercising and avoid playing sports. You often need all of your energy to survive days of pain and exhaustion. You may fear sapping your minute supply of energy and fear letting down playing partners. Experts emphasize, however, that the sick need to learn the particular exercises that match their abilities and needs. Learning just what exercise and play is possible for you can free you to enjoy yourself, feel more a part of the world, and enhance your health. There will be days when you will probably not be able to play or to exercise. And there are competitive sports that for some can induce stress. It is important to know and accept yourself. But the fact that you will sometimes be unable to participate should not be grounds for stopping play and exercise altogether.

Stress caused by threat readies our bodies for "fight or flight." Anger or fear affects the adrenal system, pumping hormones that put us on alert, ready for action; however, frequently action, for instance attacking a boss who has embarrassed us or a spouse who has hurt us, would lead to greater stress. Still, the body is ready for action—play, running hard provides that release and dissipates the stress.

A thirty-eight-year-old woman diagnosed with Lyme disease said,

> My exercise class is my pressure valve. I can go in tight, down, angry, or depressed and after a half-hour workout, I'm washed out. It's like a catharsis. I hate it when I have to miss the class.

You need to know your limits. Lack of exercise and play, which ICI may seem to dictate, leads to pent-up emotions and further fatigue.

Yoga and Stretching Exercises   Tension, sickness, and lack of exercise result in shortened, contracted muscles, tendons, and ligaments. In this condition muscles do not function easily or well. There is restricted rather than supple movement, which can lead to more tightening and to tiredness. Longer muscles with greater stretch capability are stronger, function with less energy, and relax more readily. Yoga stretching exercises or positions encourage the relaxation of these muscles.

"Yoga" comes from the Sanskrit word meaning union and derives from the teachings of Lord Krishna. It is a system of physical and spiritual development that has been handed down for thousands of years. Its ultimate goal is enlightenment and self-realization. The form of yoga practiced most often today in the West is Hatha yoga and is practiced for relaxation, greater flexibility, and release of muscle tension. The exercises have become part of calisthenic and physical therapy programs. You have seen dogs or cats stretch, especially after sleeping. Humans tend naturally to do the same thing. When we are tight or tense, we tend to stretch. If you will perform a series of exercises at a set time, perhaps at the start of your day, you will begin to feel less tense and more supple. Books abound on yoga or other exercises. A physical therapist can show you exercises matched to your particular areas of tension. Too many of us look and move as though we were years older than we are. In contrast, it is always a pleasure to see an older person moving fluidly and gracefully. Stretching every day can help the ICI patient to overcome the stress-related contracted state of muscles and, by increasing his range of motion, enable him to have a body which is youthful, graceful, and energetic.

In addition to providing greater flexibility of body, yoga can be a pathway to self-knowledge and to inner peace. Mikelle Terson, a fascinating and lovely young woman who teaches yoga in New York, reflected for us on yoga's power.

> Our ego mind distorts reality because it tries to control what it sees by judging or seeing through preconceived ideas of what we think the moment should be. The ego mind is the mind of fear; it tries to control because it fears the unknown. In yoga, one learns to trust the pauses, to faithfully enter the silence, to be completely open to what is. This place of openness and stillness allows us to see honestly and clearly and from this place of clarity we can respond consciously and make choices that are aligned with our heart and spirit. It enables us to see with a deeper "knowing" eye. Through a deeper sense of physical and mental relaxation, and through greater

self-awareness, we find a richer, more loving connection to ourselves.

Muscle Relaxation   In 1986 at Turnberry, Scotland, Gregg Norman was leading the British Open after three rounds. That evening Jack Nicklaus, a long time idol and friend of Norman's, stopped at his table in the dining room to wish him well and to give a word of advice. The next day, Norman played brilliantly and won the open. When he was asked what Nicklaus had advised he responded, "Jack told me to make sure that I lighten my grip on the club."

It's easy for us to be unaware of how we tighten up when we are anxious and under stress. One of the values of doing muscle relaxation exercises is that you can become more aware of the mind-body connection in your daily living. Notice when loud music is turned off how your shoulders tend to relax; they had tightened without any conscious decision on your part. At this moment are your legs relaxed as you read? Is your back straight and comfortable? Is your neck tight? Are your facial muscles furrowed or relaxed? Being aware of neuromuscular states can be very helpful in combating tension and staying as relaxed as possible.

There are many books that can guide you in muscle relaxation. The object is to develop awareness of your muscles in their tightened and relaxed conditions and to learn control over these muscles. The technique usually involves repeatedly tightening and loosening muscles. Usually, you are instructed to start with the muscles farthest from your head—toes, ankles, then whole foot, and so on, working your way up through all the muscles in your body until finally you complete the exercise with a focus on your facial muscles.

Learning to relax your muscles is another step to self-awareness and to greater control of your mind and your body. God knows, the stresses of ICI can tighten your whole system, but with awareness and some focus you can, as the expression says, "hang loose."

Biofeedback   Another means of coming to know ourselves and gaining greater control is biofeedback. Biofeedback is the feeding back of biological signals to the cause of
the biological activity. Under stress, when feeling fear or
anxiety, we can experience sweaty palms, dry mouth, rapid
pulse, flushed or pale skin, excessive salivation, or inability
to swallow. These are all biofeedbacks—signals from our
body that we are suffering stress. In *New Mind, New Body,*[2]
Barbara Brown says that biofeedback is an "interaction with
the interior self. It is another source of self-knowledge."
   Biofeedback has three phases:

1. body sensations recorded and measured by electrical
   equipment
2. personal awareness of the tensions and thoughts, feelings, and images causing tension
3. control of tension by choice of new images

The equipment used to record and measure stress signals are
of three kinds. An electromyograph (EMG) measures muscle tension, an EEG-like machine measures brain waves, and
a cardiovascular machine reports heart rate. By reading the
electrical feedback, you can become aware of the degree of
stress you are registering at that particular moment. Finally,
you can learn to control your stress by forming images conducive to a more relaxed state of being. Picturing a baby
sleeping or waves lapping onto the shore might help you to
release tension. If so, you would see your heart rate slow or
your brain waves change or muscular activity relax on the
biofeedback equipment.
   The purpose of biofeedback is greater self-knowledge and
self-control. The equipment can heighten your awareness of
the tension present in your body. You can then learn to
control your thoughts and images to produce a greater state
of relaxation.

Nutrition   Despite the health consciousness of our age and
the amount of leisure time that is ours to enjoy, many of us

poison our bodies with non-nourishing foods and our minds and hearts with toxic activities. If we are to feel as well as we can, we need a healthy diet for body and soul.

Annemarie Colbin, author of *Food and Healing,* insists that "there is no one diet that is right for everyone all the time." One man's meat can literally be another man's poison. Colbin writes, "It is crucial that each person contemplating a change in diet monitor his or her own body's feedback, feelings it emits of okay or not okay."[3] Even in the way that we eat, we need to know ourselves. We need to learn which foods give us energy and which contribute to our feeling sick. We have an enormous variety of foods to choose from— we need to learn to make healthy choices.

Most nutritionists agree on some basic concepts regarding the food we eat. They urge that the food we eat be natural, as much as possible in season and grown locally, that it consist of whole grains, dried legumes, fresh vegetables and fruits, fish and fowl, and for sweeteners fruit juices and maple or rice syrup. They warn against sugar, milk products, canned and frozen foods, and red meats. They encourage more carbohydrates and less fat. And they advise that the diet be balanced. As Jane Brody says in her book on nutrition, "Currently our balance is greatly distorted: Americans eat too much fat, too much sugar, too many calories, and even too much protein."[4]

Individuals with ICI need all the help that a good diet can provide. Their bodies are buffeted by pain and drained by fatigue. Unfortunately, their doctors seldom advise them to eat in a healthy way. Robert S. Mendolsohn, M.D., author of *Confessions of a Medical Heretic,* states, "Patients are increasingly aware of the aphorism that when it comes to nutrition, a doctor knows as much as his secretary—unless she has been on a diet, in which case she knows more."[5] It is easy to become so obsessed with eating properly that food becomes a source of stress rather than a relaxing, nourishing pleasure. Approached with a light heart, though, eating in a healthy manner can be a great source of needed energy and refreshment. The soul requires nourishment just as the body does if it is to maintain a healthy state. Often we fail to meet our needs for solitude, for intellectual stimulation, for artistic enjoyment. Many of our clients have come to realize how little time they take for themselves to read, to reflect, to pray. Their lives are hectic, and they are filled with guilt if they sit down to read, walk in the woods, or dangle their feet in a stream. Most of them live less than an hour from New York City; yet, out of fear or habit they do not delight themselves with ballet, theater, art, music. And though TV films or programs could enlighten and enrich them, their TV diet too often consists of fare bereft of depth or intelligence. An intelligent fifty-year-old woman who suffers from a number of infirmities told us after going to a symphony to which she had been given tickets,

> I felt totally taken out of myself and filled with wonder. The music seemed to enter all of me and give me such joy. It could have gone on all night. I know I must do things like that more often, but I fear that I won't.

Gerard Manley Hopkins said, "The world is charged with the grandeur of God."[6] We need to look into flowers, look at the night sky, visit the mountains, and cherish the trees in our back yards. We need to listen to wise words and to laugh at funny ones. Nourishment is all around us, but too often we starve ourselves in the midst of plenty.

A ninety-nine-year-old nun, a wonderful, dear friend of ours, calls us to recommend a book she has just read and to ask for suggestions. Sister Elizabeth still asks us what plays and movies she should see when she is in New York. She also always runs up stairs "for exercise" and does needle-point to "keep my fingers nimble."

Thoreau wrote

> I went to the woods because
> I wished to live deliberately,
> to front only the essential
> facts of life, and see if I

> could not learn what it had to
> teach, and not, when I came
> to die, discover that I had not
> lived.[7]

Meditation and Self-Hypnosis

> When I am particularly fatigued, I find it useful to go
> into a trance for my thirty-minute train ride; then I'm
> ready for the evening's activities.

A successful editor in New York who suffers from
migraines wrote those words describing self-hypnosis as her
way of releasing tension and tapping new energy. Many
others find meditation, particularly Transcendental Meditation, a source of rest and creativity. Robert Roth, author
of *Transcendental Meditation,* writes, "During the TM technique, the mind settles down to a silent, yet fully awake
state of awareness. At the same time the body gains a unique
and profound state of rest and relaxation."[8]

Transcendental meditation and self-hypnosis are based on
the belief that deep rest eliminates stress. As Shakespeare
put it,

> Sleep that knits up the raveled sleeve
> . . . sore labor's bath,
> Balm of hurt minds[9]

Like sleep, meditation offers very deep rest to the mind and
then to the body. In doing so, it taps a reserve of creativity
and serenity deep within the mind. Just as in sleep, physio-
logical functions—heart rate, breathing, brain waves—slow
down during deep relaxation.

If you are interested in learning to meditate, there are many
books like Robert Roth's to guide you. But if you wish to
learn the simple techniques of Transcendental Meditation,
it is necessary to attend an instructional course given by a

TM center. These courses tend to entail a four-day training workshop.

Learning to quiet your mind, to take its focus off ego-centered and often anxiety-producing thoughts, is an important goal. As we have indicated in Chapter 10 we believe that the way you think affects the way you feel, which governs the way you live. You can learn to discipline the way you talk to yourself and you can learn to give your mind periods of rest through meditation and self-hypnosis.

THE NEED TO ACHIEVE

> The happy people are those who are producing something; the bored people are those who are consuming much and producing nothing.[10]

The person with ICI is threatened by, and therefore experiences stress around, the fear of not being able to achieve all that she might desire. Janet, a lively young woman suffering with lupus, described a common plight:

> I go to bed with a clear plan of what I'm going to do the next day: put my winter clothes away, get a lot of stuff to the cleaners, join a friend for lunch—then I wake up the next morning and right away I know that, considering how I'm feeling, I can't do any of it. It's so damn frustrating.

Fatigue and pain are awful to endure, but the threat that they pose to the need to achieve is worse. As a lovely woman with MS put it,

> I can stand the pain. It's the fatigue that I can't stand, because then I can't do anything.

It takes enormous patience, self-knowledge, and wisdom to realize what you can do and to live to the fullest within those limits. Focusing on what you can't do or attempting to do what on that day you are not capable of causes terrible stress and unhappiness. Learn to have mild activities in reserve for bad days. Learn to be honest with friends and colleagues about the limitations imposed by your illness. If the truth will set you free, denying that truth will shackle you to stress, self-pity, and your illness.

THE NEED TO BE UNDERSTOOD

Individuals with ICI find themselves hungering deeply for understanding. Being misunderstood, not really listened to, results in feelings that range from frustration and irritation to aching loneliness and helpless rage. Unlike needs that you can meet for yourself, such as healthy eating habits, being understood depends on someone else's capacity for empathy. This kind of dependency can contribute to a sense of helplessness.

Meeting your needs to be heard and understood is more in your control than you might realize, however, and being misunderstood might have more to do with your expectations and behavior than you are aware. Win, a sensitive, no-nonsense nurse, described her own sense of helplessness in trying to be close to a dear friend who has fibromyalgia.

> She just cuts me out when her illness flares up. It's like she leaves me to enter a world of her own that I'm not allowed to enter.

We don't know Win's friend, but we see too many clients with a tendency to withdraw into illness, pulling curtains down on their world of friends and family. Reasons for choosing isolation vary ("No one wants to hear complaints," "I don't want pity," "How could anyone understand?"), but the result is the same—the need to be understood is unmet.

Listening with understanding is a very difficult skill, especially when the person trying to listen has many needs and feelings connected to what he is hearing. If you want to be understood, understand this difficulty. You need and deserve to be heard in what you are experiencing and what you are feeling. But what you share might make it very difficult for someone who cares for you to listen. The spouse of a woman with fibromyalgia complained,

> She says I don't listen to her, but how am I supposed to react when she says things like "I'm not going back to Dr. X. or to any other doctor," or "I can't live another year like this"?

Try to share your feelings and needs in the way we discussed in Chapters 17 and 18. As much as you might want to cry out remarks like the ones quoted above, these words veil the real feelings, for example, discouragement, anger, or fear, and trigger alarm rather than empathy in the person whose understanding you need. Understanding helps to relieve stress; lack of understanding causes it. Help those you want to hear you by your own understanding of them and your own growth in the ability to share yourself clearly.

THE NEED TO BE SUPPORTED

> I hate asking for help. I've taken pride in being self-supporting. For me, the worst thing about having lupus is needing help.

This woman's difficulty is common to most of us. It is easier to give than to receive. It is humbling to admit that we cannot do something we could once do. Growing old gracefully demands such humility—so does being sick. The individual with ICI will suffer enormous stress if she will not admit her need for support and then be assertive about getting that need met. Housecleaning, child care, shopping, or some work responsibilities might have to be done by others. You are probably very graceful in giving; learn to be graceful in receiving. Trust that others want to help, often need to help, and sometimes need to realize that they must help. Grow in appreciation of yourself, not only valuing yourself for what you can accomplish but learning with the blind poet Milton that "they also serve who only stand and wait."[11]

THE NEED TO BE LOVED

The greatest threat to our well-being—and therefore, the greatest stress—is not feeling lovable. ICI makes feeling lovable difficult. With ICI you don't feel well, you don't think that you look well, you can't accomplish what you once could, and often you feel on the outside of a healthy, normal world looking in. In addition, you are often viewed with skepticism and treated with impatience.

Against the threat of self-doubt and self-dislike, you need to believe in yourself, value yourself, love yourself.

> I bring no doctrine, I refuse to give advice, and in an argument I immediately back down. But I know that today many are feeling their way tentatively, not knowing what to put their trust in. To them I say: Believe those who seek the truth, doubt those that find it, doubt everything, but don't doubt yourself.[12]

To accomplish this goal of self-affirmation, you must drink in trust, believe the love, care, and respect of those around you. This could be your most severe challenge. You might have to pray with the young man in Scripture, "I believe, O Lord, help my unbelief" (Mark 9:24).

Faith requires not just belief in God but belief that you are of infinite worth, made in His image and likeness. You are loved and you are lovable. Avoid those whose own problems restrict them from loving you; open yourself to those who help you to believe.

THE NEED TO LOVE

"Love your neighbor as yourself."

Very often, sadly, if we loved our friends and family the way we love ourselves, they would receive pretty shoddy treatment. We tend to be less caring of ourselves than of those around us. At the same time, the less we value ourselves, the harder it is to share ourselves in love with others. But it is a basic human need to love; if that need is not met, the organism suffers stress.

ICI can turn you in on yourself, as you conserve your energy and nurse your pain. Self-care is essential, but if it results in withdrawal from the persons you love, the effect will be stressful loneliness. This loneliness can, in turn, lead to further focus on your ailments, until your life is circumscribed by an almost obsessive preoccupation with your body, its functions and malfunctions.

A junior high school teacher who has been diagnosed with colitis expressed his need to reach outside himself to care.

> I would sink without the kids. I can feel terrible in the morning. I really fear that I can't make it but I get to school and despite the pain I get involved and love it. The kids keep me from feeling sorry for myself.

Loving others, caring for their needs, brightening their lives, surprising them, delighting them, gives our own life meaning. A middle-aged woman, Harriet, who is frequently depressed by her undiagnosed fatigue condition, told us,

> When I'm down, I always call someone who I think would appreciate hearing from me. I don't complain about my condition, I tell them that I was thinking about them and wanted to say hello. I get off the phone feeling better and feeling that I've done something worthwhile for someone.

To give of yourself in the way that Harriet does requires that you value yourself and trust that a word from you could delight someone. You might find that hard to believe, but if you take the risk to give, you will begin to realize that you do have the power within you to raise someone's spirits, to make his or her day lighter.

Charity is supposed to begin at home, but loving those closest to us is the greatest challenge. Listening beneath the words to the feelings and needs of your spouse, son, daughter, friend, mother, father is a daily discipline that calls for selfless maturity. Responding with understanding rather than reacting defensively can lead to inner freedom and even wisdom.

Giving of yourself, your feelings, hopes, and dreams, despite fears of misunderstanding and rejection, builds the kind of intimacy that relieves the stress of isolation. You need to believe in yourself enough to give of yourself. You will be easing your own stress as you listen to others.

THE NEED TO BE YOURSELF

Fearing that we are not special enough or not lovable enough, we tend to play roles. If you don't trust that you will be noticed for being yourself, then maybe being "nice" or "always available" or "subservient" or "diffident" will win approval. You can learn roles in childhood and play them through life: responsible son, peace-maker daughter, good girl. Such roles squelch dimensions of yourself and therefore put you under stress.

A very charming and attractive twenty-eight-year-old named Carla who has Lyme disease told us what an eye-opener it was to discover the role she has played.

> When we moved into Tom's mother's house, I began having anxiety attacks—terrifying experiences in which I felt myself losing all control, all sense of myself. I tried to describe what was happening to me to my doctor, who gave me some medication. But only after getting into therapy did I see that I had let my mother dominate me all my life and then I had done the same with my husband. Only when we moved in with his mother did I start losing it. I couldn't stay nice and cooperative any-

more, but I didn't know any other way, so I started losing it. Now, thank God, I've learned to assert myself with Tom, my mother, and his. I have to work at it, but it feels so good. The worrying about what others will think is much less. I haven't felt the anxiety for weeks.

The organism is in stress if it cannot be itself. The song sung years ago by Sammy Davis points to the need to reject roles that interfere with being authentic so as to relate effectively: "I've gotta be me. I can't be right for somebody else, if I'm not right for me."

You have to identify roles that you play that can keep you from being free, from being authentic, and from discovering who you really are. You risk being vulnerable in shucking off old ways of acting. But you risk being stifled with stress in continuing to be less than who you really are.

Knowing ourselves, accepting ourselves, being ourselves is not easy. Approval that is given to us for role playing does not reach our hearts, it does not nourish us or help us to affirm ourselves. When we don't like ourselves, we rely on praise and try desperately to avoid blame—a recipe for stressful dependence. Regardless of illness and all its diminishments, you need to accept yourself, grow daily to appreciate yourself, and be committed to be yourself. "This above all, to thine own self be true." Trust yourself, listen to your feelings and needs, grow to understand those around you. Your illness is a daily trial, but in learning to live with it, you can come to know yourself and live a full, wise, and courageous life.

Notes

PART 1

Epigraph, Robert F. Murphy, *The Body Silent* (New York: Norton, 1990).

CHAPTER 1

Epigraph, Henrietta Aladjem, *In Search of the Sun: How to Cope with Chronic Illness* (New York: Macmillan, 1988).

CHAPTER 2

Epigraph, Mortimer Adler, in an interview with Bill Moyers, "Teaching the Constitution," WNET, New York, April 30, 1987.

1. "The CFIDS Chronicle," *Journal of the CFIDS Association* (Summer/Fall 1990), p. iii.

2. *Kalamazoo Gazette,* May 3, 1984, p. 7.

3. Beth Ediger, *Coping with Fibromyalgia* (Dallas: The Fibromyalgia Association of Texas, 1991), p. 14.

4. Ibid.

5. Peter A. Banks, Daniel H. Present, and Penny Steiner, eds., *The Crohn's Disease and Ulcerative Colitis Fact Book* (New York: Scribners, 1983), p. 3.

6. Elaine F. Shimberg, *Relief from Irritable Bowel Syndrome* (New York: M. Evans, 1988).

7. Diana Benzaia, "Lyme Disease," *Health* (June 1989), p. 73.

8. Polio Society brochure.

9. Katharina Dalton, *Once a Month* (Claremont, Calif.: Hunter House, 1987), p. 17.

CHAPTER 3

Epigraph, Alex Ward, "TV's Tormented Master," *New York Times Magazine* (November 13, 1988), p. 38.

1. Linda Crabtree, Executive Director of CMT International.

CHAPTER 4

Epigraph, William Shakespeare, *Romeo and Juliet,* III, v, 101.

1. Douglas A. Grossman, in Elaine F. Shimberg's *Relief from IBS,* (New York: Claremont, Calif.: M. Evans, 1988), p. xv.

2. Mary Lou Ballweg, *Overcoming Endometriosis: New Help from the Endometriosis Association.* (NY: Congdon and Weed, 1987), p. 3.

3. "The CFIDS Chronicle," p. iv.

4. C. Orian Truss, *The Missing Diagnosis* (N.p. 1982), p. 3.

5. Ellen Idler, *New York Times,* March 21, 1991.

6. Geoffrey Cowley with Mary Hager and Nadine Joseph, "Chronic Fatigue Syndrome," *Newsweek* (November 12, 1990).

7. Ibid.

8. "The CFIDS Chronicle," p. iii.

9. Robert M. Bennett, "Fibrositis, Does It Exist and Can It Be Treated?" *The Journal of Musculoskeletal Medecine* (June 1984).

10. Shimberg, *Relief from Irritable Bowel Syndrome.*

11. Dalton, *Once a Month,* p. 2.

12. Cowley with Hager and Joseph, "Chronic Fatigue Syndrome," p. 64.

13. William Shakespeare, *Romeo and Juliet,* III, v. 101.

CHAPTER 5

Epigraph, Mary Lou Ballweg, *Overcoming Endometriosis: New Help from the Endometriosis Association* (New York: Congdon and Weed, 1987).

1. F. C. Shontz, *The Psychological Aspects of Physical Illness and Disability,* (New York: Macmillan, 1975), p.112.

CHAPTER 6

Epigraph, Rainer Rilke, "Letters to a Young Poet."

1. Robert Soll and P. B. Grenoble, *Multiple Sclerosis: Something Can Be Done and You Can Do It* (Chicago: Contemporary Books, 1984), p. 20.

CHAPTER 7

Epigraph, Aleksandr Solzhenitsyn, *One Day in the Life of Ivan Denisovich.*

1. Arthur Kleinman, *The Illness Narratives: Suffering, Healing, and the Human Condition* (New York: Basic Books, 1988).

2. Henri Baruk, *Patients Are People Like Us* (New York: William Morrow, 1978), p. 136.

3. Daniel Goleman, *New York Times,* November 13, 1991.

4. Ibid.

CHAPTER 8

Epigraph, Mary C. Richards, *Centering* (Middletown, Conn.: Wesleyan University Press, 1962).

PART II

Epigraph, Rose Kennedy.

CHAPTER 9

Epigraph, Pablo Casals, *Joys and Sorrows: Reflections by Pablo Casals as Told to Albert E. Kahn* (New York: Simon and Schuster, 1970), p. 295.

CHAPTER 10

Epigraph, Author unknown, "Desiderata," found in St. Paul's Church, Baltimore, 1692.

1. John 8:32.

2. Aaron T. Beck and Gary Emery with Ruth L. Greenberg, *Anxiety Disorders and Phobias* (New York: Basic Books, 1985), p. 63.

3. Albert Ellis, *Reason and Emotion in Psychotherapy* (Secaucus, N.J.: Citadel Press, 1962).

CHAPTER 11

Epigraph, The Beatles, "Let It Be" (from the album *Let It Be,* New York, Apple Records).

1. Aaron T. Beck, *Love Is Never Enough* (New York: Harper & Row, 1988).

2. William Shakespeare, *Hamlet* I, iii, 75.

CHAPTER 12

Epigraph, William Wordsworth, "I Wandered Lonely as A Cloud."

1. Arnold Lazarus, *In the Mind's Eye* (New York: Rawson Associates, 1977).

CHAPTER 13

Epigraph, William Shakespeare, *As You Like It,* II, vii, 139.

CHAPTER 14

Epigraph, Dietrich Bonhoeffer, *The Cost of Discipleship* (New York: Macmillan, 1966), p. 19.

1. Sam Keen, "Your Mythic Journey with Sam Keen," Interview with Bill Moyers, WNET, New York, April 15, 1991.

2. Ibid.

3. Michael White and David Epston, *Narrative Means to Therapeutic Ends* (New York: Norton, 1990), p. 30.

CHAPTER 15

Epigraph, Anatole Broyard, "Doctor Talk to Me," *New York Times Magazine,* August 26, 1990.

1. Carl R. Rogers, Unpublished presentation at the Summer Institute of the Center for the Studies of the Person, La Jolla, California, 1968.

2. J. D. Salinger, *Franny and Zooey* (Boston: Little, Brown, 1961), p. 109.

3. Thomas L. English, "Skeptical of Skeptics," *JAMA* 265, no. 8 (February 27, 1991), p. 964.

4. Broyard, "Doctor Talk To Me."

5. Ibid.

CHAPTER 16

Epigraph, Michel Eyquem de Montaigne, "Essais," as quoted by Gail Goodwin in *Mother and Two Daughters* (New York: Viking Press, 1982).

1. Daniel Goleman, *New York Times,* April 27, 1989.

2. William Shakespeare, Sonnet 116, "Let Me Not to the Marriage of True Minds."

3. Bernard Gunther and Corita Kent, *High Cards, Picture Poem Post Cards* (New York: Harper & Row, 1974).

CHAPTER 17

Epigraph, Dinah Criak, an eighteenth-century poet.

CHAPTER 18

Epigraph, Carl R. Rogers, "Some Elements of Effective Interpersonal Communication," Unpublished talk at the California Institute of Technology, Pasadena, November 9, 1964.

1. Sidney Jourard, *The Transparent Self* (New York: D. Van Nostrand, 1971), p. 6.

CHAPTER 19

Epigraph, Simon and Garfunkel, "The 59th Street Bridge Song," from the album *Parsley, Sage, Rosemary, and Thyme,* New York, Columbia Records.

1. T. Schwartz, "Making Waves: Can Dr. Irv Dardik's Therapy Really Work Miracles?" *New York* (March 18, 1991).

2. Barbara Brown, *New Mind, New Body* (New York: Harper & Row, 1974).

3. Annemarie Colbin, *Food and Healing* (New York: Ballantine Books, 1986), p. xiv.

4. Jane Brody, *Jane Brody's Nutrition Book* (New York: Norton, 1981), p. 5.

5. Robert S. Mendolsohn, *Confessions of a Medical Heretic,* as quoted in Colbin, *Food and Healing,* p. xiii.

6. Gerard Manley Hopkins, "God's Grandeur," in *The Poems of Gerard Manley Hopkins,* edited by W. H. Gardner and N. H. Mackenzie (London: Oxford University Press, 1976), p. 66.

7. Henry D. Thoreau, "Walden Pond."

8. Robert Roth, *Transcendental Meditation* (New York: Donald I. Fine, 1987), p. 7.

9. William Shakespeare, *Macbeth,* II, ii, 36.

10. Dean Inge, as quoted in Rabbi Samuel Silver, *How I Enjoy This Moment* (New York: Trident Press, 1967), p. 113.

11. John Milton, "On His Blindness."

12. André Gide, . . . *La Séquestrée de Poitiers* (Paris: Gallimard, 1930).

Authors' Recommended Reading List

Aladjem, H. *In Search of the Sun: How to Cope with Chronic Illness*. New York: Macmillian, 1988.

Henrietta Aladjem's personal story of her battle with lupus, an excellent example of someone dealing with a chronic illness.

Beck, A. T. *Love Is Never Enough*. New York: Harper & Row, 1988.

The father of cognitive psychology applies his insights to help couples overcome misunderstanding and resolve conflicts.

Bonhoeffer, D. *The Cost of Discipleship*. New York: Macmillan, 1963.

Bonhoeffer was a brilliant young German theologian put to death by the Nazis. His book is a powerful analysis of the challenge of being a Christian in the modern world.

Ellis, A. *A New Guide to Rational Living*. North Hollywood, Calif.: Wilshire, 1975.

This book discusses the irrational thoughts that we repeat to ourselves and that keep us troubled. It points the way to feeling better by thinking more rationally.

Frankl, V. E. *Man's Search for Meaning*. New York: Washington Square Press, 1963.

A psychiatrist who learned after three years at Auschwitz that his entire family had been wiped out writes about mankind's search for a higher meaning in life.

Jourard, S. M. *The Transparent Self*. New York: D. Van Nostrand, 1971.

Jourard's thesis is that we pay a great price for camouflaging our real selves in an effort to avoid criticism and rejection. We come to know ourselves as we reveal our true selves to someone we can trust.

Keen, S. *To a Dancing God*. New York: Harper & Row, 1970.

A delightful book, poetic and theological, that explores the problems of being genuine in a changing world. Keen discusses with humor and insight faith, education, sexuality, and personal storytelling.

Kushner, H. S. *When Bad Things Happen to Good People*. New York: Avon, 1981.

A rabbi writes from the agony of watching his fourteen-year-old son die of a rare disease. He asks "Why?" and then answers with wisdom, faith, and love.

Lazarus, A. A. *In the Mind's Eye*. New York: Rawson Associates, 1977.

A profound discussion of the role that images play in our lives.

Missiline, E. H. *Your Inner Child of the Past*. New York: Pocket Books, 1982.

Missiline stresses the need to discover the child we once were to see how this child has power over our adult lives.

Morrow-Lindberg, A. *A Gift from the Sea*. New York: Pantheon, 1955.

The wife of Charles Lindbergh takes the reader with her on a reflective, retreat-like vacation. She considers the pressures and distractions of a busy life.

Peck, S. *The Road Less Traveled*. New York: Simon and Schuster, 1978.

Peck states that life is difficult and so is changing that life. He describes the road to growth and to peace as the process of confronting our problems honestly.

Richards, M. C. *Centering*. New York: Wesleyan Press, 1962.

Mary Catherine Richards uses the image of centering clay on a potter's wheel to reflect poetically and deeply on the process of centering one's life.

Rogers, C. R. *A Way of Being*. Boston: Houghton Mifflin, 1980.

Carl Rogers has been an inspiration to us. His last book is a reflection on the way of being that he attempted to study and to live.

Strong, M. *Mainstay: For the Well Spouse of the Chronically Ill*. New York: Penguin Books, 1988.

In a frank and touching manner, Strong describes the experience of herself, her husband, and their children in dealing with her husband's multiple sclerosis.

Tannen, D. *You Just Don't Understand*. New York: Ballantine Books, 1990.

This book, though written by a linguistics expert, demonstrates in an interesting and clear way the differences between male and female in communication. It is a valuable book for spouses and others in intimate relationships to read together.

Teilhard de Chardin. *The Divine Milieu*. New York: Dodd, Mead, 1983.

A brilliant priest-scientist meditates on his conviction that God can be seen everywhere in the world. It is a profound and inspiring book written by a saintly genius.

Tillich, P. *The Shaking of the Foundation*. New York: Scribners, 1948.

A collection of the theologian's psychological sermons. Our favorite is "You are Accepted."

Van Kaam, A. *Religion and Personality*. New York: Prentice Hall, 1964.

A theological–psychological study of the development of a healthy personality that attempts to integrate religious beliefs with personal growth.

General Reading List
on Illnesses

Aladjem, H. *In Search of the Sun: How to Cope with Chronic Illness.* New York: Macmillan, 1988.

———. *Understanding Lupus.* New York: Scribners, 1985.

Armstrong, A. *A Breath of Life.* London: British Broadcasting, 1985.

Arnold, C. *Pain: What Is It? How Do We Deal with It?* New York: Morrow, 1986.

Ballweg, M. L. *Overcoming Endometriosis: New Help from the Endometriosis Association.* New York: Congdon and Weed, 1987.

Banks, P. A., Present, D. H., and Steiner, P. *The Crohn's Disease and Ulcerative Colitis Fact Book.* New York: Scribners, 1983.

Bender, S. D., and Kelleher, K. *A Positive Program to Pain Control.* Tucson: Body Press, 1986.

Benzaia, D. *Protect Yourself from Lyme Disease: The New York Medical Guide to Prevention, Detection, and Treatment.* New York: Dell, 1989.

Berland, T. *Living with Your Colitis and Hemorrhoids and Related Disorders.* New York: St. Martin's Press, 1975.

Blau, S. P., and Schultz, D. *Lupus: The Body Against Itself.* New York: Doubleday, 1984.

Brandt, L. J., and Grossman, P. S., eds. *Treating IBD: A Patient's Guide to the Medical and Surgical Management of Inflammatory Bowel Disease.* New York: Raven Press, 1989.

Breitkopf, L. J. *Coping with Endometriosis.* New York: Prentice Hall, 1988.

Dalton, K. *Once a Month.* Claremont, Calif.: Hunter House, 1987.

————. *The Original Premenstrual Syndrome Handbook.* Claremont, Calif.: Hunter House, 1990.

Dudley, R., and Rowland, W. *How to Find Relief from Migraine.* New York: Beaufort Books, 1982.

Ediger, B. *Coping with Fibromyalgia.* Dallas: The Fibromyalgia Association of Texas, 1991.

Feiden, K. *Hope and Help for Chronic Fatigue Syndrome.* New York: Prentice Hall, 1990.

Foley, K. M., and Payne, R. M. *Current Therapy of Pain.* Toronto, B.C.: Decker, 1989.

France, R. D., and Krishnan, K. R. *Chronic Pain.* Washington, D.C.: American Psychiatric Press, 1988.

Franklin, M., and Sullivan, J. *The New Mystery Fatigue Epedemic: What Is It? Have You Got It? How to Get Better.* New York: Random House, 1990.

Goldstein, J. A. *Could Your Doctor Be Wrong?* New York: Pharos Press, 1991.

Hallpike, J. F., Adams, C. W., and Tourtelotte, W. W., eds. *Multiple Sclerosis: Pathology, Diagnosis, and Management.* Baltimore: Williams and Wilkins, 1983.

Harrison, M. *Self-Help for Premenstrual Syndrome.* New York: Random House, 1985.

Hawkridge, C. *Understanding Endometriosis.* London: MacDonald, 1989. Published in conjunction with the National Endometriosis Society, Great Britain.

Hoffman, R. L. *Seven Weeks to a Settled Stomach: Free Yourself from Digestive Pain Forever with the Hoffman Self-Help Program*. New York: Simon and Schuster, 1990.

Jacobs, G., and Kerrins, J. *The AIDS Fight: What We Need to Know About AIDs Now*. Woodshole, Mass.: Cromlech Books, 1987.

Kidd, P. M., and Huber, W. *Living with the AIDS Virus: A Strategy for Long Term Survival*. Berkeley, Calif.: HK Biomedical, 1990.

Kleinman, A. *The Illness Narratives: Suffering, Healing, and the Human Condition*. New York: Basic Books, 1988.

Lance, J. W. *Migraine and Other Headaches*. New York: Scribners, 1986.

Laureson, H. H., and de Swaan, C. *The Endometriosis Answer Book: New Hope New Help*. New York: Rawson Associates, 1988.

Laureson, and Stikans, E. *Premenstrual Syndrome and You: Next Month Can Be Different*. New York: Simon and Schuster, 1983.

Laurie, G., Maynard, F. M., Fischer, D. A., and Raymond, J., eds. *Handbook on the Late Effects of Poliomyelitis for Physicians and Survivors*. St. Louis, Mo.: Gazette International Networking Institute, 1984.

Lawrence, R. M. *Goodbye Pain! Two Dozen Ways You Can Prevent and Relieve Pain*. Santa Barbara, Calif.: Woodbridge Press, 1989.

Lechtenberg, R. *Multiple Sclerosis Fact Book*. Philadelphia: F. A. Davis, 1988.

Lipton, S., Tunks, E., and Zoppi, L., eds. *The Pain Clinic: Advances in Pain Research and Therapy*. Vol. 13. New York: Raven Press, 1990.

Lovelace, R., and Shapiro, H., eds. *Charcot-Marie-Tooth Disorders: Pathophysiology, Molecular Genetics, and Therapy*. New York: Wiley-Liss, 1989.

Matthews, W. B. *Multiple Sclerosis: The Facts*. New York: Oxford University Press, 1985.

Milam, L. W. *The Cripple Liberation Front Marching Band Blues*. San Diego: Mho Mho Works, 1984.

Norris, R. V., and Sullivan, C. *PMS: Premenstrual Syndrome.* New York: Rawson Associates, 1983.

Older, J. *Endometriosis.* New York: Scribners, 1984.

Pentajan, J. H. *Multiple Sclerosis Handbook for Patients-Family-Physicians.* Salt Lake City: Utah Chapter National Multiple Sclerosis Society, 1980.

Permut, J. B. *Embracing the Wolf: A Lupus Victim and Her Family Learn to Live with Chronic Disease.* Atlanta: Cherokee, 1989.

Phillips, R. H. *Coping with Lupus: A Guide to Living with Lupus for You and Your family.* Wayne, N.J.: Avery, 1984.

Pitzele, S. K. *We Are Not Alone: Learning to Live with Chronic Illness.* New York: Workman, 1987.

Podell, R. N. *Doctor, Why Am I So Tired?* New York: Pharos Press, 1987.

Register, C. *Living with Chronic Illness: Days of Patience and Passion.* New York: Free Press, 1987.

Rose, F. C., and Gawel, M. *Migraine: The Facts.* New York: Oxford University Press, 1989.

Rosner, L. J., Ross, S. *Multiple Sclerosis: New Hope and Practical Advice for People with MS and Their Families.* New York: Prentice Hall, 1987.

Scala, J. *Eating Right for a Bad Gut: The Complete Nutritional Guide for Ileitis, Colitis, Crohn's Disease, and Irritable Bowel Syndrome.* New York: New American Library, 1990.

Scanlon, D., and Becnel, B. C. *The Wellness Book of Irritable Bowel Syndrome: A Guide to Lifelong Relief from the Symptoms of the Most Common and Least Talked About Ailment, IBS.* New York: St. Martin's Press, 1989.

Scheinberg, L. C., ed. *MS: A Guide for Patients and Their Families.* New York: Raven, 1983.

Shimberg, E. F. *Relief from Irritable Bowel Syndrome.* New York: M. Evans, 1988.

Shontz, F. C. *The Psychological Aspects of Physical Illness and Disability.* New York: Macmillan, 1975.

Shuman, R., and Schwartz, J. *Understanding Multiple Sclerosis: A Guidebook for Families*. New York: Scribners, 1988.

Silverstein, A., and Silverstein, V. *Lyme Disease, the Great Imitator: How to Prevent and Cure It*. Lebanon, N.J.: AVSTAR, 1990.

Sloan, I. J. *AIDS Law: Implications for the Individual and Society*. New York: Oceana, 1988.

Soll, R. W., and Grenoble, P. B. *Something Can Be Done and You Can Do It: A New Approach to Understanding and Managing Multiple Sclerosis*. Chicago: Contemporary Books, 1984.

Sternbach, R. A. *Mastering Pain: A Twelve Step Program for Coping with Chronic Pain*. New York: Putnam, 1987.

Thompson, W. G. *Gut Reaction: Understanding Symptoms of the Digestive Tract*. New York: Plenum Press, 1989.

Tollison, C. D. *Managing Chronic Pain: A Patient's Guide*. New York: Sterling, 1984.

Weinstein, K. *Living with Endometriosis: How to Cope with the Physical and Emotional Challenges*. Reading, Mass.: Addison-Wesley, 1987.

Whitmore, G. *Someone Was Here: Profiles in the AIDS Epidemic*. New York: New American Library, 1988.

Witt, R. L. *PMS: What Every Woman Should Know About Premenstrual Syndrome*. New York: Stein and Day, 1983.

Illness Associations

We encourage you to join the association of your illness. By joining, you help to support the search for cure and appropriate treatments. The association provides information on the illness, its course, current research, and the latest effective treatments. Many of the organizations maintain a list of support groups in the United States and Canada. Each association provides a list of literature regarding the illness—books, pamphlets, brochures, magazine articles, medical journal articles—that can be purchased at low fees.

Contact with people who are trying to deal with the same illness with which you are suffering can be very comforting. We are deeply impressed with the courage, determination, and commitment of the people who organize and maintain these organizations.

AIDS Clinical Trials Information Service
PO Box 6421
Rockville, MD 20849-6421
(800) TRIALS-A
(800) 874-2572
(800) 243-7012 (Deaf Access)
Manager: Sue Herbert
Services: ACTIS is a central resource that provides current information on federally and privately sponsored clinical trials for AIDS patients and others infected with the HIV.

American Association for the Study of Headache
875 Kings Highway
Suite 200
West Deptford, NJ 08096
(609) 845-0322
(609) 384-5811 (FAX)
Executive Director: Robert K. Talley
Services: AASH is a professional organization for MDs, DDs, nurses, and PhDs. Its objectives are: to promote the exchange of ideas about the cause and treatment of headache; to provide education for professionals and laity; to encourage scientific studies in the treatment of headache; to develop and provide educational materials.

American Autoimmune Related Diseases Association
Michigan National Bank Building
15475 Gratiot Avenue
Detroit, MI 48205
(313) 371-8600
(313) 371-6002 (FAX)
President and Executive Director: Virginia T. Ladd
Services: Provides public forums, physician symposia, free informational materials on autoimmune diseases, peer support groups, referrals, and research support.

American Chronic Pain Association, Inc.
PO Box 850
Rocklin, PA 95677
(916) 632-0922
(916) 632-3208 (FAX)
Executive Director: Penney Cowan
Services: Provides self-help, peer support, and coping skills for anyone with chronic pain. More than 800 chapters worldwide.

American Diabetes Association
1660 Duke Street
Alexandria, VA 22314
(703) 549-1500
(703) 836-7439 (FAX)
Vice President of Communications: Jerry Franz
Services: The mission of the American Diabetes Association is to prevent and cure dia-

betes and to improve the lives of all people affected by diabetes.

Arthritis Foundation

1314 Spring Street, NW
Atlanta, GA 30309
(404) 872-7100
(800) 283-7800
(404) 872-0457 (FAX)
President: Don L. Riggin
Services: Seeks to discover cause and improve the methods for treatment and prevention of arthritis and other rheumatic diseases, to increase the number of scientists investigating rheumatic diseases, and to educate the public.

Association De La Fibromyosite Du Quebec

11 Rue Dorius
Repentigny, Quebec
Canada J6A 4X9
(514) 582-3075
President: Marguerite-Rose Pesant Bedard
Services: Provides support and information for people with fibromyalgia.

Bay Area Lupus Foundation

2635 North First Street
Suite 206
San Jose, CA 95134
(800) 523-3363
(for California)
(408) 954-8600

Executive Director: Jo Dewhirst
Services: Maintains library of medical articles; publishes quarterly newsletter; provides information and referral in English and Spanish; conducts and presents educational series; provides free public screening and testing for lupus. 17 subchapters throughout northern California.

Celiac Sprue Association/ USA

745 North 58th Street
Omaha, NE 68132-2003
(402) 558-0600
(402) 558-1347 (FAX)
Executive Director: Leon H. Rottmann
Services: Provides information and referral services for patients with nontropical sprue and dermatitis herpetiformis, details on the gluten-free diet, a quarterly newsletter, *Lifeline,* and related handbooks and literature. 74 chapter groups and 38 resource units serve six regions of the U.S.

The CFIDS Association of America, Inc.

PO Box 220398
Charlotte, NC 28222-0398
(800) 44-CFIDS
(704) 365-9755 (FAX)
Executive Director: Kim Kenney

Services: Publishes a quarterly chronicle; provides local referral for support groups and health-care professionals; funds CFIDS research and advocacy efforts.

Charcot-Marie-Tooth Association
601 Upland Avenue
Upland, PA 19015
(610) 499-7486
(800) 606-CMTA
(610) 499-7487 (FAX)
Office Administrator: Patricia Dreibelbis
Services: Publishes a quarterly newsletter; organizes regional patient-family conferences; makes physician referrals; provides support group referrals. 30 support groups.

CMT International: Charcot-Marie-Tooth Disease Peroneal Muscular Atrophy International Association, Inc.
One Springbank Drive
St. Catharines, Ontario
Canada L25 2K1
(416) 687-3630
Executive Director: Mrs. Linda Crabtree
Services: Publishes a bimonthly newsletter; organizes biennial convention; conducts regional meetings featuring

free clinics; offers counseling. 6 regional chapters internationally.

Crohn's & Colitis Foundation of America
386 Park Avenue South
17th Floor
New York, NY 10016
(212) 685-3440
(800) 932-2423
(212) 779-4098 (FAX)
National Executive Director: Barbara Boyle
Services: Funds research to find a cure for Crohn's disease and ulcerative colitis; provides educational programs for patients, medical professionals, and the general public; offers supportive services for patients and their families and friends. 97 chapters.

Digestive Disease National Coalition
711 Second Street NE
Suite 200
Washington, DC 20002
(202) 544-7497
(202) 546-7105 (FAX)
Washington Representative: Dale P. Dirks
Services: Provides patient education brochures.

Endometriosis Association
International Headquarters
8585 North 76th Place

Milwaukee, WI 53223
(414) 355-2200
(414) 355-6065 (FAX)
(800) 992-3636
President: Mary Lou Ballweg
Services: Provides support for women with endometriosis and families affected by it, support groups listing, crisis call helpers, direct individual assistance; publishes *Overcoming Endometriosis: New Help From the Endometriosis Association*. 75 chapters and support groups.

Exceptional Cancer Patients
300 Plaza Middlesex
Middletown, CT 06457
(860) 343-5950
Co-Director: Tim Albaitis
Services: Provides support and education to people with chronic or life-challenging illnesses.

Fibromyalgia Association of British Columbia
PO Box 15455
Vancouver, BC
Canada V6E 129
(604) 688-0503
President: Judith Verstick
Services: Publishes membership newsletter; provides disability information; lobbies the government; hosts educational forums for people with fibromylagia; maintains fibromyalgia information data base. 19 support groups.

Fibromyalgia Association of Central Ohio
PO Box 21988
Columbus, OH 43221-0988
(614) 457-4222
President: Mary Anne Saathoff
Services: Organizes support meetings; maintains a library of information, including articles, videotapes, and audiotapes.

Fibromyalgia Network
PO Box 31750
Tucson, AZ 85751-1750
(520) 290-5508
(520) 290-5550 (FAX)
Owner/Publisher: Kristin Thorson
Services: Primary service is a quarterly newsletter; also provides patients with over 75 self-help group contacts in the United States and Canada, physician referrals, and other information pertaining to fibromyalgia.

International Polio Network
4207 Lindell Blvd., #110
St. Louis, MO 63108-2915
(314) 534-0475
(314) 534-5070 (FAX)

Executive Director: Joan L. Headley
Services: Provides information on polio and its late effects; provides referrals; publishes a quarterly newsletter and handbook on the *Late Effects of Poliomyelitis for Physicians and Survivors*; lists clinics, health professionals, and support groups; coordinates periodic international conferences; encourages research and the exchange of information among related groups.

Interstitial Cystitis Association

PO Box 1553
Madison Square Station
New York City, NY 10159
(212) 979-6057
(212) 677-6139 (FAX)
President: Vicki Ratner
Executive Director: Debra Slade
Services: Provides patients with up-to-date information on interstitial cystitis; provides support; educates the medical community.

Intestinal Disease Foundation

1323 Forbes Avenue
Suite 200
Pittsburgh, PA 15219
(412) 261-5888
(412) 471-2722 (FAX)
Executive Director: Linda

Schorr
Services: Provides support and information for people with chronic intestinal disease and conditions, phone support, and educational materials about conditions such as irritable bowel syndrome, Crohn's disease and ulcerative colitis; publishes quarterly newsletter.

Lupus Foundation of America, Inc.

1300 Piccard Drive
Suite 200
Rockville, MD 20850-4303
(301) 670-9292
(800) 558-0121
(301) 670-9486 (FAX)
Executive Director: John M. Huber
Services: Provides patient information, referrals to chapter support groups, and physician referral services; contributes to public awareness. 100 chapters.

Lupus Network, Inc.

230 Ranch Drive
Bridgeport, CT 06606
(203) 372-5795
President: Linda J. Rosinsky
Services: Publishes a newsletter, *Heliogram*, which explores orthodox and unorthodox information concerning lupus and other autoimmune diseases. Limited literature reprints.

Lyme Disease Foundation
1 Financial Plaza
18th Floor
Hartford, CT 06103
(860) 525-2000
(860) 525-TICK
Executive Director: Thomas
E. Forschner
Services: Provides educational material, patient support, legislative action, and physician referrals; funds research.

Myasthenia Gravis Foundation of America
222 South Riverside Plaza
Suite 1540
Chicago, IL 60606
(312) 258-0522
(800) 541-5454
(312) 258-0461 (FAX)
Executive Director: Anna El-Qudsi
Services: Dedicated to the detection, treatment, and cure of myasthenia gravis; provides lay and professional material.

National AIDS Clearinghouse
PO Box 6003
Rockville, MD 20849-6003
(800) 458-5231
(800) 243-7012 (TTY/TDD-Deaf Access)
(301) 738-6616 (FAX)
Project Director: Ruthann Bates
Services: Specialists answer the toll-free number and answer inquiries, make referrals, help locate publications pertaining to HIV infection and AIDS.

National AIDS Hotline
PO Box 13827
Research Triangle Park, NC 27709
(800) 342-2437 (Hotline)
(919) 361-4622
(919) 361-7889 (TTY/TDD-Deaf Access)
(919) 361-5736 (FAX)
Administrative Manager: Catherine Stuart
Services: Provides confidential information and referrals and free written materials. A toll-free service of the U.S. Department of Health and Human Services, the Public Health Service, and The Centers for Disease Control.

National Chronic Fatigue Syndrome and Fibromyalgia Association
3521 Broadway
Suite 222
Kansas City, MO 64111
(816) 931-4777
(816) 753-6706 (FAX)
President: Orvalene Prewitt
Services: Sponsors educational programs; maintains speakers bureau; provides hotline.

National Chronic Pain Outreach Association, Inc.
7979 Old Georgetown Road
Suite 100
Bethesda, MD 20814
(301) 652-4948
(301) 907-0745 (FAX)
President: William E. Hurwitz, MD
Director: Doug Ventura
Services: Provides educational material; produces quarterly newsletter, *Lifeline,* which focuses on pain management methods and coping skills, as well as positive personal experiences and book reviews.

National Digestive Diseases Information Clearinghouse
2 Information Way
Bethesda, MD 20892-3570
(301) 654-3810
(301) 907-8906
Director: Kathy Kranzfelder
Services: Provides information about digestive diseases to the public, patients and their families, and physicians and other health care providers. A congressionally mandated service of the National Institute of Diabetes and Digestive and Kidney Diseases of the National Institutes of Health.

National Family Caregivers Association
9621 East Bexhill Drive
Kensington, MD 20895-3104
(301) 942-6430
(800) 896-3650
(301) 942-2302 (FAX)
President: Suzanne Mintz
Administrative Manager: Diane Walden
Services: Provides caregiver-to-caregiver support network; a guide, *The Resourceful Caregiver,* and newsletter, *Take Care!.*

National Graves' Disease Foundation
320 Arlington Road
Jacksonville, FL 32211
(904) 724-0770
Executive Director: Nancy H. Patterson, Ph.D.
Services: Facilitates establishment of support groups for members in all states; fosters public awareness and education on the causes, effects, and treatments of Graves' disease.

National Headache Foundation
428 West St. James Place
2nd Floor
Chicago, IL 60614-2750
(800) 843-2256
(312) 525-7357 (FAX)
Director: Suzanne E. Simons
Services: Serves as an information source to headache sufferers, their families, and the physicians who treat them;

promotes research into and offers free information on potential headache causes and treatments; educates the public.

National Multiple Sclerosis Society

733 3rd Avenue
New York, NY 10017
(212) 986-3240
(800) Fight-MS
(212) 986-7981 (FAX)
President: General Michael Dugan
Services: Provides counseling, education, information, referrals, and general assistance to those affected by multiple sclerosis; public policy advocacy. 140 chapters and branches.

National Organization for Rare Disorders

PO Box 8923
New Fairfield, CT 06812-8923
(203) 746-6518
(203) 746-6481 (FAX)
President: Abbey S. Meyers
Services: Clearinghouse of information for those wishing to learn about rare disorders; networking; advocacy; referrals to resources.

National Self-Help Clearinghouse

25 West 43rd Street
Room 620
New York, NY 10036
(212) 354-8525
(212) 642-1956 (FAX)
Executive Director: Audrey Gartner
Services: Provides information and referral to self-help support groups, technical assistance in starting and maintaining self-help groups; publishes a newsletter.

National Sjögren's Syndrome Association

PO Box 42207
Phoenix, AZ 85080-2207
(602) 516-0787
(800) 395-6772
(602) 516-0111 (FAX)
Executive Director: Barbara Henry
Services: Promotes public awareness of Sjögren's syndrome; encourages research into the cause and cure of the disorder.

National Vulvodynia Association

PO Box 19288
Sarasota, FL 34276-2288
(941) 927-8503
(941) 927-8602 (FAX)
Communications Director: Marjorie MacArthur
Services: Membership provides support groups, patient advocacy, and research on this

difficult-to-diagnose gyneco-
logical disorder.

National Women's Health Network

514 10th Street, NW
Suite 400
Washington, DC 20004
(202) 347-1140
(202) 347-1168 (FAX)
Executive Director: Beverly
Baker
Services: An advocacy non-
profit organization giving
women a greater voice in the
health-care system; monitors
health-related regulatory
agencies and reviews proposed
federal legislation; publishes a
bimonthly newsletter.

North American Chronic Pain Association of Canada

150 Central Park Drive
Suite 105
Brampton, Ontario
Canada L67 2T9
(905) 793-5230
(800) 616-7246
(905) 793-8781 (FAX)
President: Dr. Ric Edwards
Services: Forms local support
groups for those who suffer
chronic pain; trains sufferers as
leaders of the support groups.
A volunteer organization of 39
chapters; an affiliate of American Chronic Pain Association.

Ontario Fibrositis Association

250 Bloor Street East
Suite 401
Toronto, Ontario
Canada M4W 3P2
(416) 967-1414
*Project Development
Administrator:* Robin
Saunders
Services: Provides informa-
tion regarding support, cop-
ing, and learning about fi-
bromyalgia. 22 chapters.

People With AIDS Coalition

50 W 17th Street
8th Floor
New York, NY 10011-1607
(212) 647-1415
(800) 828-3280
(212) 447-1508 (FAX)
Executive Director:
Christopher L. Babick
Services: Provides people affected by AIDS with information to enable them to make
well-educated choices; promotes the philosophy and
practice of self-empowerment
that will ultimately improve
the quality of life.

The Polio Society

4200 Wisconsin Avenue
Suite 106273
Washington, DC 20016
(301) 897-8180
(202) 466-1911

Options *Editor:* Jessica Scheer
Services: Provides state-of-the-art medical and psychological information to polio survivors, their families, friends, and physicians; produces a quarterly newsletter, *Options*; sponsors monthly information/support group meetings and patient-oriented conferences.

Scleroderma Federation
Peabody Office Building
1 Newbury Street
Peabody, MA 01960
(508) 535-6600
(800) 422-1113 (Hotline)
(508) 535-6696 (FAX)
President: Marie Coyle
Services: Provides literature, quarterly newsletter, *The Beacon*, local support groups, helpline, peer counseling, physician referrals, emotional support group meetings, and educational meetings.

Scleroderma International Foundation
704 Gardner Center Road
New Castle, PA 16101
(412) 652-3109
President: Arkie Barlet
Services: Provides a supportive network for individuals with the disease; supports research into the cause, cure, and control of scleroderma; strives

to educate patients, physicians, and public.

Sjögren's Syndrome Foundation
333 North Broadway
Suite 2000
Jericho, NY 11753
(516) 933-6365
(800) 475-6473
(516) 933-6368 (FAX)
Executive Director: Rita M. May
Services: Publishes the newsletter *The Moisture Seekers* and *The Sjögren's Syndrome Handbook*; provides a network of chapters, groups, and resource volunteers throughout the U.S. and Canada, professional and patient symposia, and funding for meritorious research.

Society for Menstrual Cycle Research
10559 N 104th Place
Scottsdale, AZ 85258
(602) 451-9731
Secretary-Treasurer: Mary Anna Friederich, MD
Services: Goals are: to identify research priorities; recommend research strategies; promote interdisciplinary research on the menstrual cycle.

The Thyroid Foundation of America, Inc.

Ruth Sleeper Hall 350-
RSL350
40 Parkman Street
Boston, MA 02114-2698
(617) 726-8500
(800) 832-8321
President: Lawrence C.
Wood, M.D.
Services: Provides health education and support for thyroid patients and health care
professionals; promotes public
awareness of thyroid problems; raises and distributes
funds for thyroid research.

United Scleroderma
Foundation

PO Box 399
Watsonville, CA 95077-0399
(408) 728-2202
(800) 722-HOPE
(408) 728-3328 (FAX)
Executive Director: Nancy
Wemp
Services: Establishes and
maintains support networks;
encourages medical research to
find the cause and cure for
scleroderma and related colla-
gen diseases.

USA Fibrositis
Association

PO Box 20408
Columbus, OH 43220
(614) 764-8010
CEO: Burt D. Miskimen
Services: Underwrites and
cosponsors research projects;

finances local activities in support of fibromyalgia; organizes and finances seminars;
sponsors delegates to national
meetings.

Vestibular Disorders
Association

PO Box 4467
Portland, OR 97208-4467
(503) 229-7705
(503) 229-8064 (FAX)
Services: Provides educational material; produces
newsletter; educates public
and health professionals about
vestibular disorders; provides
a support network for people
and families affected by dizziness and balance disorders.

The Well Spouse
Foundation

610 Lexington Avenue, Rm. 814
New York, NY 10022
(212) 644-1241
(800) 838-0879
FAX: (212) 644-1338
Executive Director:
Patricia Aldrich Still
Services: Provides support
groups and emotional support
to spouses of the chronically
ill; raises consciousness of professionals to the plight of the
well spouse; advocates for legislative changes in insurance
coverage for respite care; produces a bimonthly newsletter,
WSF Newsletter.

Index

abandonment, fear of, 35
abdominal pain, 21, 22, 27
acceptance, of disease, 30, 32, 34–35, 43,
    52–53, 55–56, 61, 70, 76, 77, 78,
    104, 107–8, 148, 181, 240
    see also adjustments, emotional and
        physical; coping
achievement, need for, 234–35
acne, 27
acting out, of feelings, 172, 176, 178,
    194, 204
action, positive, 226
ACTIS (AIDS Clinical Trials Informa-
    tion Service), 257–58
active listening, 209
activities, curtailment of, 32, 58–68, 97–
    98, 135–36, 182–84
acute stress, described, 224–25
adjustments, emotional and physical, 55–
    71
    automatic thinking and, 108, 110
    case histories of, 55–56, 58, 60–61
    courage and, 43, 52–53, 55–56, 61, 70,
        146, 148, 181, 240
    diagnostic confirmation in, 68–71
    to exacerbations, 59–64, 103, 138–39,
        181–82
    humility and, 157, 167, 168, 236
    to remissions, 64–66, 103, 182
    as severely taxing, 66–68
    uncertainty and, 12, 32, 67–68
    see also acceptance, of disease; coping;
        self-help strategies, realistic
Adler, Mortimer, 12
advice, well-meaning, 171, 178–79, 208,
    211, 223
aggressive rage, 54
aging, as rationalization, 32
AIDS, 19–20, 52–53, 148
    see also HIV infection
AIDS Clinical Trials Information Service
    (ACTIS), 257–58
AIDS-related complex (ARC), 19
Aladjem, Henrietta, 3, 33, 132
alcohol, 22, 109

allergies, 12
alpha-delta sleep disruption, 18
ambiguity, of symptoms, 67–68
    see also diagnoses
American Association for the Study of
    Headache, 258
American Chronic Pain Association,
    Inc., 258
American Hospital Association, 84
American Lupus Society, 258
ampligen, 71
anemia, 23
anger, 30–31, 109, 123, 146, 148
antibiotics, Lyme disease and, 24
anxiety, 29, 34, 178, 179
    in anticipating future, 32, 97–104, 122,
        129–39, 182–184
    automatic thinking and, 106
    distraction technique and, 99
    irrational imagery and, 135
    see also fear
apologies, 30
appearance, reality of illness vs., 4–6, 12,
    14, 39, 42, 62–66, 89–90, 91
appetite, loss of, 21, 22, 24
approval, role-playing for, 239, 240
ARC (AIDS-related complex), 19
arched foot, 15
arthritis, 24
Association De La Fibromyosite Du
    Quebec, 258–59
associations, ICI, 47, 148, 257–68
attitude, positive control of, 77
aura symptoms, 24
authentic behavior, *see* honesty, of feel-
    ings; responsibility
automatic thinking, 105–15
    anxiety and, 106
    awareness of, 108, 110, 122, 124, 125,
        128, 133, 135
    case histories of, 106, 108–9
    decisions based on, 106–7, 108
    programmed ineffective action and,
        109–10
    as self-serving, 144